Improving Care for Veterans Facing Illness and Death

Edited by Kenneth J. Doka & Amy S. Tucci

Foreword by Chuck Hagel, U.S. Secretary of Defense

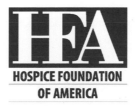

HOSPICE FOUNDATION OF AMERICA

This book is part of Hospice Foundation of America's *Living with Grief®* series.

Rich Otto

© 2013 Hospice Foundation of America®

This book is part of HFA's Living with Grief® series.

Ordering information:

Call Hospice Foundation of America: 800-854-3402

Or write:
Hospice Foundation of America
1710 Rhode Island Avenue, NW #400
Washington, DC 20036

Or visit HFA's Web site:
www.hospicefoundation.org

Managing Editor: Lisa McGahey Veglahn
Layout and Design: The YGS Group

Publisher's Cataloging-in-Publication
(Provided by Quality Books, Inc.)

Improving care for veterans facing illness and death /
    edited by Kenneth J. Doka and Amy S. Tucci; foreword by Chuck Hagel.
    p. cm.
    Includes bibliographical references and index.
    LCCN 2012952554
    ISBN 9781893349162

    1. Veterans--Medical care--United States.
    2. Terminal care--United States.   I. Doka, Kenneth J.
    II. Tucci, Amy S.

    UB369.I47 2013   362.86'0973
                     QBI13-600006

Dedication

To our veterans and their families

For service and sacrifice

Contents

Acknowledgments i

Foreword
Chuck Hagel iii

PART I:
THE MILITARY EXPERIENCE 1

1. The Military Milieu: A Grin-and-Bear-It Culture
   Deborah Grassman 3

2. *Voices*: Understanding the Military Culture as a Context for Delivering
   Hospice Care: A Practical Application
   Deborah Grassman 19

3. The Military Mindset
   James Hallenbeck 25

4. *Voices*: Why Didn't Anyone Ever Ask?
   David Abrams 39

5. Generational Cohorts: A Military Perspective
   Kenneth J. Doka 47

PART II:
SPECIAL ISSUES IN TREATING VETERANS AT THE END OF LIFE .. 55

6. History of Hospice and Palliative Care in the
   Department of Veterans Affairs
   James Hallenbeck 59

7. Coping with Trauma and Posttraumatic Stress Disorder (PTSD) at
   Life's End: Managing Life Review
   Ryan Weller 71

8. Grief and Traumatic Stress: Conceptualizations and Counseling
   Services for Veterans
   Lori R. Daniels 85

9. Forgiveness: A Reckoning Process that Facilitates Peace
   Deborah Grassman 95

10. *Voices*: A Voice From a Clinician
    Deborah Grassman 105

11. Special Issues in Pain Management
   V.S. Periyakoil..111

12. *Voices*: The Survivalist. Or Tired and Brave.
   Nicky Quinlan 127

13. Caring for Seriously Ill Veterans in the Community: Communication,
   Collaboration, and Coordination
   Diane H. Jones..133

14. Programs that Work: *We Honor Veterans*..149

PART III:
GRIEF AND LOSS...157

15. Sacred Ceremonies, Sacred Space: The Role of Rituals and Memorials
   in Grief and Loss
   Kenneth J. Doka..161

16. Profaning the Sacred: The Disruption of Military Funerals
   Kenneth J. Doka..171

17. Serving the Bereavement Needs of Veterans and Their Families
   Patricia McGuire 175

18. Combat Death: A Clinical Perspective
   Jill Harrington-LaMorie with Betsy Beard..................................189

19. *Voices*: A Military Widow
   Joanne Steen..213

20. Military Suicide: Counseling Survivors
   Antoon A. Leenaars 219

Concluding Comments
   Kenneth J. Doka..241

RESOURCES 243

INDEX 247

Acknowledgments

It is our tradition to begin by thanking the small staff of the Hospice Foundation of America, consisting of Spencer Levine, Kristen Baker, and Lindsey Currin. It amazes us how much this small staff accomplishes. We are sure it amazes them as well.

We also thank a supportive board of directors for all their efforts. Special recognition goes to our managing editor Lisa McGahey Veglahn, who kept us on deadline and carefully reviewed all aspects of production.

This year, we offer a special thanks to the Department of Veterans Affairs (VA). They have been so much a part of the process, suggesting and securing authors. We want to offer a special thanks to Scott Shreve and Deborah Grassman. Not only did they suggest authors but they made us aware of documents in the public domain, such as the Department of Veterans Affairs *2011 Hospice and Palliative Care Annual Report*, which was so helpful.

Naturally we also need to thank all the authors who responded to tight deadlines. Both editors would like to thank their families and friends for their patience as we worked to publish a complex book in such a short time. You know who you are!

As always, we wish to recognize the continuing legacy of the late Jack Gordon, founder and former chair of Hospice Foundation of America (HFA); Myra MacPherson, board member and advisor; and David Abrams, former HFA president, current board member, always friend, and this year a *Voices* author.

Foreword

Chuck Hagel

The character of a nation is judged by many things, including how it cares for its veterans. That care requires a completeness of understanding of veterans, their experiences, their lives, their families, their fears, and their needs. Too often we approach these human challenges and needs with a clinical mindset and tone. Veterans' care requires a full universe of understanding of their lives and the complexities of those lives. This is noticeably true for veterans dealing with Posttraumatic Stress Disorder (PTSD), some of whom are now needing end-of-life care, as well as younger veterans facing re-entry problems in a society that does not always understand.

The Hospice Foundation of America (HFA), as it celebrates 20 years of comforting and wonderful work, has recognized these unique issues for veterans. HFA has been effective and relevant because of its educational outreach to institutions and individuals, helping them more fully understand these human dimensions. The broader the understanding of veterans by caregivers, the more comfort we can give to our veterans and their families. We must remember that families are an integral part of caregiving; families are usually the centerpiece of a veteran's life.

All human beings deserve dignity in their lives, especially at the end. And there is no group of Americans more deserving of this dignity than veterans. All who work with, live with, respect, and love veterans know this. They also know that veterans never have expected special privileges or see themselves as better as or more special than other citizens. Their sacrifices were made because they felt and lived a sense of purpose greater than their own self-interest. This point is so important when working with and caring for veterans. In the end all any of us have are our faith, family, and friends… and our dignity.

Like most Vietnam veterans, my brother, Tom, and I saw a lot of combat in Vietnam during our 1968 tour. We sent five Purple Hearts and a Bronze Star home to our mother. Tom and I were fortunate, but we saw fellow soldiers who were not and others who returned with emotional and physical problems. Our hearts go out to any veteran and their families of any war, as do all Americans.

To all the selfless magnificent caregivers in our country and the world, we thank you. No one thanks you more than the veterans you serve. And no one understands better the love and respect you give them.

Chuck Hagel
U.S. Secretary of Defense

Editor's Note: U.S. Secretary of Defense Chuck Hagel agreed to write this foreword prior to his nomination by President Obama to the cabinet post. He was confirmed as Secretary of Defense as the book went to press. Hospice Foundation of America is grateful for his contribution, written and submitted to HFA before his confirmation.

The Military Experience

In recent years, Hospice Foundation of America's books and programs have focused on the challenge of how culture impacts end-of-life care. In 2009, we broadly explored the issue in *Diversity and End-of-Life Care*. Two years later, we focused on spirituality, one aspect of diversity. Other programs that dealt with cancer and end-of-life ethics were also extremely sensitive to the cultural differences that are inherent in the understanding and treatment of cancer, as well as the ways that culture and spirituality influence ethical decision making.

This year, the focus on improving care for veterans facing illness and death continues that exploration of diversity. As the opening chapters indicate, military life is a culture in and of itself, a way of life with common experiences and shared values.

Both Grassman's and Hallenbeck's opening chapters consider the unique components of military culture, or as they prefer to see it, military cultures. Both authors, in their own way and style, note the diversity of military experience. Some veterans enlist, for a multitude of reasons ranging from a paycheck to patriotism. Others were reluctantly drafted. Veterans have served in different units of the military, each with its own unique cultural nuances. They serve at different ranks and different times.

Yet despite these differences, the very nature of military experience and culture cultivates a sense of camaraderie. This camaraderie has long been noted already; in an extensive study of American soldiers in World War II, they demonstrated that loyalty to one another was the primary motivation as to why soldiers were willing to risk their lives. Fundamentally, they did so to protect their buddies (Stouffer et al., 1949). Moreover, as Grassman notes, this culture may be shared by family members such as spouses or children.

Both chapters are sensitive about that diversity, especially exploring the different receptions that met veterans as they returned from World War II, Korea, and Vietnam. Both chapters also review how the shared components of military culture and experience might influence end-of-life care.

Two issues predominate. The first is the prevailing culture of stoicism. Military culture values the forbearance of pain. As later chapters stress, this can create difficulties for pain management as veterans face illness and dying.

A second factor is the experience of combat. Soldiers often carry traumatic memories of the violence of conflict. As Hallenbeck notes, illness and death may subconsciously or consciously release these memories, creating the emergence or reemergence of symptoms of Posttraumatic Stress Disorder.

Two *Voices* pieces support this first section. Grassman's account of Arthur and Luke graphically illustrates the ways that stoicism and control may complicate end-of-life care, even as camaraderie may offer opportunities for mutual and appropriate support. Abrams' *Voices* piece reminds readers of another insidious aspect of military culture. Persons in the military may have had exposure to varied toxic agents that might impair health and complicate medical assessment and treatment. Abrams echoes a somewhat similar concern expressed by Hallenbeck, noting that an increased sensitivity from healthcare professionals to a person's possible military service can have an important impact on diagnosis and care.

Doka introduces the idea of generational differences. Different generations enter the military shaped by the unique historical, social, and demographic experiences that have framed that generation. Caregivers need to be sensitive to these generational differences, reinventing care for each cohort.

REFERENCE

Stouffer, S., Lumsdaine, R., Harper, M., Smith, M., Janis, I., Star, S., & Cottrell, L. (1949). *The American soldier: Combat and its aftermath, (V-4)*. Princeton, NJ: Princeton University Press.

CHAPTER 1

The Military Milieu: A Grin-and-Bear-It Culture

Deborah Grassman

For those who work with veterans, it is important to understand the commonalities of the military culture. There are aspects of veterans that may be different from their civilian counterparts. These differences arise from the many different factors that influence the creation of military culture. Yet there is no single, universal military culture. Veterans have served in different branches of the service; they held different ranks. Some willingly enlisted; others unwillingly enlisted; some were drafted. Some served in combat; others have not, although all were trained in combat and had to be willing to go to war if necessary. Some felt lost after discharge from service, saying something to the effect of: "I left the shelter of my family for the shelter of the military. When I got out, I looked around and said, 'Now what?' I didn't know how to go on." Other veterans say just the opposite, reporting that the military provided direction and skills that helped them define themselves.

People joined the military for different reasons. Many were motivated by patriotism: "I love this country. I couldn't think of a better way to serve than to become a soldier." Others joined for the benefits the military offered: "I love to travel. I got to see the world."

Some joined for the training and educational benefits that accompany service. Some joined to get away from situations: "I was just a pimply-faced, disobedient kid wanting to get away from home. I joined the military so I could get out on my own." Others had gotten into trouble with the law and were told they could choose between the military or jail.

Some veterans served unwillingly. One veteran said he did not want to serve, "but I wasn't smart enough to go to college to maintain a deferment. I didn't want to move to Canada to avoid the draft. I had no choice." Some served willingly, yet still suffered disappointment. One veteran said he signed up to go to Vietnam, but he was sent to join a unit in Europe instead: "I've always felt like I was only good enough to make the second-string team; I could practice with the team, but I wasn't good enough to play." Some veterans have said that they joined the military to avenge the death of a buddy killed in war.

Soldiers express a range of feelings about the training. Most say that the military was the best thing that ever happened to them: "It taught me how to grow up and become an adult." Others were ambivalent. They were not necessarily glad or proud to have served: "I was forced to participate in something I didn't believe in."

Basic training was grueling for some, but the skills they learned were essential to keeping them alive in warfare: "Each of us was mentally torn down. It wasn't until we were completely broken down that we could be rebuilt." For others, it was demoralizing: "We were taught to shut up and listen. We were told that they didn't care about what we thought; the only thing they cared about was that we did what we were told. I came out feeling that I was insignificant and that no one cared." The tactics used to create a unified military team could be harsh: "When a recruit makes a mistake, he's singled out, but everyone is disciplined for it. Individualism is poison when you're building a team-oriented fighting force. We succeed or fail together." They were taught control: "We were supposed to be perfectionists, down to the smallest detail, even in the way our shoes were shined and beds were made. The training helped us learn how to control our environment." Punishment was sometimes extreme: "Minor infractions might be met with having to clean floors and toilets with toothbrushes or exercising so vigorously we vomited."

The environment fostered camaraderie: "We would literally eat, sleep, shower, learn, laugh, cry, sweat, and bleed as a cohesive unit. All is shared and no one's ever left behind. We're taught to be our brother's keeper. The collective welfare always outweighs the needs of the individual." The risks of not being able to count on each other were high: "We were tested mentally and physically every day. It's important to find out who can adapt to difficult circumstances. Anyone who can't poses a risk. We put our lives in the hands of our leaders and comrades each day. In this way, we gave each other life, or if mistakes were made, death."

Training got rougher when "kill or be killed" instincts had to be developed: "We had to be able to kill automatically. Our lives and our comrade's lives depended on it. If you took time to think, you wouldn't pull the trigger and you'd get killed." Anger fuels instincts: "You can't kill someone you're not angry at." Training built endurance: "There are few greater sins in the eyes of a soldier than to fail or let other soldiers down. We'd rather die than fail or give up. We became more machines than humans." There were rites of passage that fostered strength: "When I was a new airman, the spiked metal wing pins were held against my chest while the other airmen pounded them until my undershirt was bloody."

Once training was completed, they sacrificed comfort: "Sometimes we lived in harsh living conditions. There were long deployments away from our family to hostile parts of the world. There was always the threat of death. And, sometimes, there was death itself." Physical scars were worn as a badge of honor: "They come with bragging rights. But emotional scars bring jeers. A soldier must be able to prove he has courage and can not only take pain, but have pride in the fact he can endure it so well. We can't show fear. Fear and pain are seen as signs of weakness. 'I can handle it' is our motto." They were taught how to live in survival mode: "In some ways, I've never come out of that mode. Some days I'm on automatic pilot, like a robot."

Some identify ambivalence with their role in society: "We bear the scars of our suffering as a badge of courage, yet we often suffer in silence. We pay the price demanded for the American way of life." Even after discharge, military service continued to exert its influence: "After I left, I lost my identity. I didn't fit in. I was straddling two worlds and didn't belong to either. I didn't even know how to settle a dispute or deal with conflicts that arose. All the rules had changed. Nothing was regulated anymore." They sometimes felt devalued: "I used to be important; other peoples' lives depended on me. Now, I'm a nobody." Some veterans have said that they became "adrenaline junkies," causing them to drive recklessly or have difficulty adjusting to mundane civilian life: "I was used to action and drama. When I got home, I was bored. I wanted adventure."

Veterans also identify the price their families paid: "I got the recognition, while my wife's sacrifices went unnoticed. She's the one who had to learn to maintain the house and car, balance the checkbook, give birth without me at her side, provide childcare alone, console lonely children, take care of family emergencies, and attend funerals. She did this for months on end, without support, often with financial hardship, while constantly worrying I would be killed and not come home." Combat veterans sometimes talk about the difficulty they have empathizing with other peoples' problems. They have seen the worst that humankind has to offer and everything else pales in comparison: "My girlfriend complained because she didn't have the right clothes to wear to a party. I got angry. I wanted to scream, 'I was a POW in Korea. Let me tell you about things to complain about.' Instead, I walked out and never returned any of her phone calls."

Children paid a price too. One adult son of a career-military soldier identifying himself as a "military brat" asked a poignant question: "Do you know how hard it was for a little boy to say good-bye to his dad every time there was a skirmish in the world? Do you know what it's like to want to watch the news more than cartoons so you can find out whether your dad is safe? Do you know how much damage was done to me every time my dad left and the adults turned to me and said, 'You're the man of the house now'?"

The Marine Corps seems to be in a category all its own with especially effective indoctrinations. "Once a Marine, always a Marine," says the slogan. They are tough; they face illness as though it were an enemy combatant. One Marine said there was a sign on their barracks: "Pain is weakness leaving the body." It explained why he did not want to take pain medication for the advanced cancer he now had. Marines' deaths can sometimes be difficult. As one veteran in hospice said, "You can't kill a Marine." Unfortunately, they do not always let go easily as they are dying.

As distinct as the military is from civilian society, it is also a reflection of society. The military gets the strong, the weak, the smart, the less-than-smart, the evil, the good, and the truly exceptional in the same proportion as the American citizenry. After induction, however, the creation of the rugged soldier who can "handle anything" starts to emerge. Like a plant's spore whose hardened shell can endure the severest weather, germinating years later, military beliefs continue to exert their influence throughout their lifespan.

Part of the reason military indoctrination is so effective is because it occurred at an impressionable age when people were forming their young-adult identity. Away from family, with a desire to belong, young men and women defined themselves within the military culture, which imprinted its belief systems at a critical stage of development. When recruits were issued a uniform, they clothed themselves in a new identity as well; remnants were often retained long after the uniform was gone.

For those working with veterans, developing an appreciation for the many difficulties soldiers experience upon returning to civilian life is important. The soldiers were used to being "out of country," and once discharged from active duty and assuming veteran status, many felt as though they remained out of country in their own country. While the rest of its citizens had been spending young adult years learning how to gain skills and knowledge to get along in the world, America's troops were learning how to *fight* the world. Their relationships were often temporary, dissolving with the next set of transfer orders. Not only were the normal growth and developmental tasks of young adulthood bypassed, but they learned a culture that focused on protection and killing, which was sometimes at odds with day-to-day living. Often they did not realize how much their experiences had changed them: "I thought I'd serve my country, come home, remove the uniform, and resume my life where I left off. I had no idea how life-changing those few years were. At that age, I was so naive."

These indoctrinated beliefs did not always yield easily to new information or civilian culture. Even when soldiers were offered the opportunity to participate in military programs to help them adjust to civilian life, the soldiers often refused because of their eagerness to return home: "I didn't want debriefing. All I wanted was to get back to my family. I'd been away long enough." Some cite inexperience that often accompanies youthful thinking: "I thought I knew everything in order to go back to being a civilian. I didn't want to listen to others telling me what I thought I already knew." Soldiers seldom learned how to let go of stoic values that kept them from themselves and the ones who loved them.

THE CULTURE OF COMBAT

Embedded within the military culture is another culture, the culture of war. Although a few soldiers were motivated for self-glorification and promotion in combat zones, most were motivated for different reasons. They did not fight for themselves; they were selflessly motivated to fight for a cause and to fight for comrades. They were willing to lay down their lives for each other. Many exhibited extraordinary acts of bravery to preserve their buddies' survival or accomplish an important mission. Yet the longer-term impact of this behavior was not always positive. Many soldiers sustained emotional, mental, social, spiritual, and moral injuries that sometimes caused a lifetime of suffering. This suffering can often be kept submerged in unconsciousness, but at the time of death, wartime memories sometimes emerge unbidden.

As is true overall with military culture, combat culture is not universal. Each war was different. Each had its own culture that exerted a different influence on young soldiers, and it is essential that professional caregivers understand these differences.

World War II was enthusiastically supported by Americans. Some veterans joined the military when they were as young as 14, lying about their ages so they could fight. Virtually everyone sought a way to support the war effort. Citizens grew victory gardens and the Red Cross sent pictures of the gardens to the soldiers so they could see their country's support. Women worked in munitions factories while others stayed home and made clothing for the soldiers. No one was left untouched.

Without televisions, the public could be shielded from war's brutality. War could be glamorized, which increased its appeal and fostered national unity. The mission of World War II enhanced this unity; it was clear and largely undisputed, especially after the bombing of Pearl Harbor. The soldiers knew they were in the war for its duration. This fostered cohesion and a determination to get the mission accomplished, a "we're in this together until the job gets done" attitude. When the war was over, troops came home together. They were greeted as heroes by a public eager to hear their victorious wartime stories.

While the adulation was gratifying, the soldiers needed more from their friends, families, and the media. They had been through horrors they could not have imagined; they had done things they never thought they would do. They needed the approval they were getting, but they also needed to give voice to the traumas they had suffered. The waiting public, however, only wanted to hear about acts of bravery and heroism, not of trauma and moral confusion. The soldiers themselves often downplayed their acts of courage: "The real heroes were those that didn't come home" or "I was just doing my duty." This kind of reticence was sometimes taken for modesty, but some veterans say that it was not modesty. They did not feel like heroes because they knew the ugly, despairing, or cowardly acts of war: "If you knew what I did, you wouldn't think I was so heroic." These stories often remained untold, lurking in the veterans' consciousness; they often hid guilt and shame.

The Korean War was different. Known later as the "Forgotten War," it was never an officially declared war; rather, it was called a "conflict" or "police action." There were no ticker tape parades for these returning soldiers; during the 1950s, people wanted to forget about war and focus more on growing prosperity. Korean veterans' trauma had been minimized or neglected and their combat contributions sometimes forgotten. For these reasons, Korean War veterans are often more reluctant to discuss their experiences or even claim their status as a veteran.

If Korea taught the American public how to ignore soldiers, Vietnam taught the public how to shame and dishonor them. There was extensive television coverage from Vietnam. Americans now understood the brutality of war, and many were at odds with its politics. Protests were organized across college campuses.

Many young men had mixed feelings about the Vietnam War, and some opposed it. The draft forced these and others into military service and then into combat. Imposed beliefs from fathers who were World War II veterans sometimes prompted unwilling sons to volunteer for Vietnam. Some sons sought the hero status their World War II fathers had held in the family (and usually came back disappointed).

These soldiers often became more cynical after their experience in Vietnam, and their cynicism affected the soldiers who believed the war was necessary. This prevailing mood is depicted by a caption on a painting by Dale Samuelson in the National Vietnam Veterans Art Museum in Chicago. It reflects the bitterness that corrodes the souls of some veterans.

We the willing
Led by the unknowing
Do the necessary
For the ungrateful

In addition to political influences, there were pragmatic factors. Although they could volunteer for more, soldiers were required to do only one-year tours in Vietnam. Rather than the "we're in this together until we get the job done" attitude of World War II soldiers, they tended to think in terms of "rotating through until my tour's up." Reports of antiwar protests at home shook their confidence in the war as well.

Frequently rotated new troops also meant fewer available seasoned troops: "You couldn't trust new soldiers to cover your back." Green recruits were also more trigger-happy: "They were more likely to kill our own soldiers who they mistook as enemy soldiers." This is known as "friendly fire."

War tactics also varied in different wars. Before Vietnam, there was a certain level of safety "behind the lines" (if there can be any safety in a war), which allowed a small degree of mental and emotional recuperation between battles. In Vietnam, however, it was guerilla warfare. There was no safe place to let defenses down, no "front lines" to fight behind. The enemy easily infiltrated, making it difficult for soldiers to distinguish friend from foe. Soldiers were on guard even in their sleep. Explosives were sometimes hidden on dead bodies, blowing up when soldiers came to retrieve them. Commonly, soldiers would carry food on them so they could give it to village children, but this could be used against them. Sometimes, the children were booby-trapped to explode while in the soldiers' midst.

As important as any of the military factors was how the public treated Vietnam veterans. Unlike World War II veterans, these men and women were not welcomed as heroes. Often they were not welcomed home at all. Antiwar protests had grown and many people who had advocated bringing the soldiers home now turned their anger against the soldiers themselves. Protesters greeted returning soldiers at the airports by spitting on them and shouting "baby killers" or "murderers." As a result, soldiers often hid their history about Vietnam like a dirty secret.

Americans did not like to feel they had "lost" the war, even when it may not have had anything to do with the warriors. The public did not want to hear about Vietnam; they wanted no reminders. As a result, soldiers' stories had nowhere to go. They could not even talk with each other much of the time. Unlike World War II soldiers who often came home in boats or trains that gave them time to share their experiences and debrief along the way, Vietnam soldiers were flown home into a hostile civilian culture in a single day. Their suffering was never validated; their souls were left burdened and their stories left untold because the public did not want to listen.

World War II veterans rightfully swell up with pride when Adolf Hitler is mentioned. "We got him," they will say, feeling the satisfaction of being part of a successful campaign to protect the world from evil. Vietnam veterans rarely feel this kind of satisfaction. Uncertainty and ambiguity about the goals and outcomes of the war often erode any sense of achieved purpose. Without a convincing victory, veterans felt their sacrifices had been meaningless. The political nature of the war added to their sense of injustice: "We could have won that war if the politicians had stayed out of it," or "They never financed the war so that we had the resources to do what needed to be done. They sent us in there knowing we couldn't win." This sense that their sufferings had been futile could linger a long time, corrupting their civilian lives and even their deaths years later.

Joining the Veterans of Foreign Wars, American Legion, or Disabled American Veterans organizations did not generally help Vietnam veterans either. They did not always feel welcome at these organizations: "They don't understand us." Even some World War II vets could not comprehend that Vietnam was different; they viewed these soldiers as "wimps" who had "lost" the war. This generational clash and culture clash interfered with communication and support. Initially, the Veterans of Foreign Wars posts did not allow Korean or Vietnam vets to even join because those wars were not "declared" wars. Although that is no longer the case, it has taken years for the American public to register more understanding and acceptance; for most Vietnam vets, the damage had already been done.

It is too soon to know how hospice care will need to be modified for veterans of more recent wars. No doubt, many factors will be the same, but some factors will be different. Another important consideration in caring for veterans is to remember that many veterans who did not serve in a declared "combat zone" have also experienced the consequences of a combat culture. Dangerous missions are required for numerous military assignments. In fact, sometimes the trauma sustained in these missions can be even more damaging because it often goes unacknowledged or is minimized. Noncombat military deaths occurred in more than 18,000 Korean-era veterans, 42,000 Vietnam-era veterans, and 2,000 Gulf War-era veterans (Department of Defense and Veterans Administration, 2012). All veterans set aside prime years in their lives, delayed personal goals, separated from loved ones, and went to strange and sometimes dangerous parts of the world. They were expected to do difficult jobs they may or may not have been inclined to perform, all the while "grinning and bearing it" or "biting the bullet." All were trained to defend their country and be willing to risk their lives if necessary to do so.

Doing a life review with hospice patients is often therapeutic. When working with veterans, including military history as part of a veteran's life review can be important. Many organizations caring for aging and dying veterans facilitate military life review by participating in the *Veterans History Project*. The mission of the project is to collect military stories directly from the veterans themselves. The hope is that future generations will "better understand the realities of war" (www.veteranshistoryproject.org).

STOICISM: AN ELEMENT OF MILITARY CULTURE THAT IMPACTS HOSPICE CARE

Webster's New World Dictionary (1995) defines the word "stoic" as "showing indifference to joy, grief, pleasure, pain." Thus, stoic people are able to disconnect from their emotional dimension. But stoic "indifference" can sometimes be experienced by others as cold, uncaring detachment.

Downplaying their suffering and feeling shame about "weak" feelings, veterans often confuse stoicism with courage. Courage is not about covering up and "putting on a good face," nor is it about "being strong" by hiding behind stoic walls. Not only is there no shame in being human, but there is freedom in being able to acknowledge that humanness and fully experience it. This acknowledgement is not a weakness; it requires strength and courage. Veterans sometime view "letting go" as admitting defeat or an act of surrender, something good soldiers do not do. Veterans often benefit from a shift in their perspective so they can see this kind of courage, the courage to encounter uncomfortable emotions openly and without apology. This shift can help them encounter feelings of sadness, fear, guilt, and helplessness that can naturally arise in the dying process. Suppressing these feelings can contribute to agitation, potentially sabotaging peaceful dying.

Stoicism is necessary, even essential, on the battlefield, but what about after the battle is over? When the soldier becomes a husband, a father, or a dying human being, the walls that stoicism erects outlast their usefulness. These walls keep out necessary feelings, and sometimes even other people. Stoicism can create protection from untrustworthy influences in anyone's life for a time; but as a long-term coping mechanism, it can be stifling. An overreliance on stoicism creates problems as serious as the problems it has been used to counteract.

Mature mental health includes identifying needs and asking for help when it is needed. Both of these actions require vulnerability. Stoicism often keeps veterans from saying what they need or allowing others to meet their needs. This mask of invulnerability sometimes may not even allow them to admit they have needs. This attitude can cause frustration, not only for themselves but also for their families or professional caregivers. Fear of vulnerability can also prevent veterans from seeking or accepting help for depression or Posttraumatic Stress Disorder (PTSD).

Stoicism might be conceptualized as having three components: pride, control, and independence. Dying is a humbling experience that challenges all of these. Control is gradually lost, pride takes a blow, and independence is eroded. Sooner or later, the stoic wall has to crumble. Later means fighting to the bitter end; sooner means a weary soldier may finally be able to surrender to hope for a peaceful death.

If a veteran cannot let go of pride, control, and independence and reach out for help, suffering might be increased. However, letting go of these qualities takes work just as creating them did. Pride can prevent veterans from acknowledging failing health, weakness, or other changes. It might mean not listening to one's own body or working beyond the point that the body is saying it is tired. Pride keeps people from seeking medical help, ignoring or belittling symptoms until it is too late to do any good. It can even keep people from admitting that they are dying. Helping veterans let go of pride allows new worlds to open.

Control increases the chance of conquering enemies on a battlefield; being vulnerable can get you killed. There is nothing like death to make people realize how little control they have. Yet, once made to realize that they are going to die, veterans sometime want to control its timing, getting angry and frustrated with the waiting. "I'm not dead and I'm not alive. If things can't go back to how they used to be, then let's get this over with now." Sometimes they even think they can control death. One veteran told his inpatient hospice team: "You shouldn't be telling patients that it's okay to die. You should be telling them to get more courage so they can get up out of these beds and fight death." This veteran had no way of knowing that peace awaits those who are able to let go of the instinct to defend and control, even though it can be so difficult to do.

Fierce independence seldom yields without a fight. "I can handle it myself" is simply not always true. Nothing is more embarrassing than for a proud and independent veteran to have to ask for help with personal needs. Nonetheless, most veterans learn to let go of control, allowing themselves to become completely human, growing in humility as they learn how to ask for help and how to become a gracious receiver, discovering connection and compassion in the process. This takes courage, and it is as heroic as facing any enemy in battle. Watching veterans grow in humility, courage, and honesty to deal with the effects of stoicism or war trauma makes working with them a true privilege.

Developing stoicism is valuable when protection is needed or unsafe environments threaten emotional harm. Stoicism can help prevent getting lost in emotions: "Time to get a backbone" or "Get a grip" or "Fake it 'til you make it" are all ways of saying, "A little stoicism might help." Thus, after suffering is validated and feelings acknowledged and felt, it is often helpful to use stoicism as a means of navigating the world. Control over putting up and letting down a stoic wall is the goal.

Carefully approaching stoic walls with veterans requires skill, art, and an understanding of military culture. Clinicians can encourage and support veterans to face their hidden feelings. But trying to coax veterans out from behind their wall of silence is not only inappropriate, it can undermine trust. Some will choose to die as stoically as they have lived, and this too needs to be respected. Many veterans, however, respond to simple, gentle invitations to allow themselves the benefit of emotional expression so that they do not use stoicism as a means of negating the validity of their own experience. Thus, the clinician's personal questions become: Can there be a way to create a safe emotional environment where letting go of stoicism can be offered without being imposed? Can the stoic wall be viewed, instead, as a door veterans can open or close at will and as often as they want, leaving the safety of their stoicism available to them? Would veterans be willing to come out from behind their walls once they experience the vitality of the released energy they had disconnected from so many years before?

MILITARY SUBCULTURE:
POSTTRAUMATIC STRESS DISORDER (PTSD)

Stoicism permeates military culture, whether a veteran served in combat or not. Combat veterans, and others who have served in dangerous-duty assignments, have to additionally cope with traumatic memories. For some, the memories crystallize into a constellation of symptoms known as Posttraumatic Stress Disorder (PTSD). Trust plays an important role in helping veterans with PTSD because these veterans do not trust easily. They have been taught not to trust. Betray a combat veteran once, and a clinician can become the enemy. These veterans can sniff out a phony instantly, so authenticity is important.

In a hospice program, trust may need to be gained quickly because the veteran may not have long to live; time to build a trusting relationship is simply a luxury that is not always available. The clinician's movements, tone of voice, and open language become important opportunities to convey trustworthiness. Additionally, people with PTSD will often "test" clinicians to see if they can be trusted. Thus, dialogues about death should be done openly and directly when a veteran with PTSD is admitted to a hospice program. Covering up "death" or "hospice" with euphemisms might trigger suspicion. These veterans faced death before when they were in combat; in fact, they were required to complete advance directives and wills whenever they went into a combat zone. Veterans are used to open dialogue about dying; they do not like "sugar coating" difficult issues and generally prefer direct language.

Some veterans with PTSD use colorful language. This, too, can be an opportunity to build trust quickly. For example, a newly admitted veteran to a hospice program might say, "I've been through a lot of shit in the last few weeks." The clinician has an opportunity to connect with the veteran by responding, "What is the most difficult shit you've had to deal with?" This helps the veteran know that the clinician is not scared of him, nor is the clinician judgmental about his language. Although it seems like a small gesture, it can go a long way to help the clinician pass the veteran's "muster test." In no way does this imply that the clinician should curse to personally express him or herself around the veteran. It simply means using the veteran's context to respond to a clinical situation because it helps trust develop more quickly.

DELIVERING HOSPICE CARE WITHIN A MILITARY CONTEXT: A SUMMARY

- Each war was different. Each had its own culture that exerted a different influence on young soldiers. Helping veterans and their families access the *Veterans History Project* can preserve military memories and promote life review.
- The value of stoicism so earnestly and necessarily indoctrinated in young soldiers might interfere with peaceful deaths for all veterans, depending on the degree to which stoicism permeated their later lives. Stoicism might also play a role in veterans' reluctance to report pain or take medications to control symptoms.
- Clinicians need to learn how to create safe emotional environments for veterans so that these veterans can let down their stoic walls. This can be done by helping veterans know that not only is there no shame in being human, but there can be freedom in being able to acknowledge and fully experience it. This is not a weakness; it requires strength and courage.
- Trust plays in important role in helping veterans with PTSD because these veterans do not trust easily. Dialogues about death should be done openly and directly upon admission to a hospice program.

Deborah Grassman, *ARNP, is a nurse practitioner. Her career at Bay Pines VA in St. Petersburg, FL, lasted for nearly 30 years, where she was the director of the hospice program. She recently retired from the VA and now provides education and consultation throughout the country. Ms. Grassman is the author of* Peace at Last: Stories of Hope and Healing for Veterans and Their Families *(Vandamere Press, 2009) and* The Hero Within: Redeeming the Destiny We Were Born to Fulfill *(Vandamere Press, 2012).*

REFERENCES

Neufeldt, V., & Sparks, A. (Eds.). (1995). Webster's new world dictionary. New York, NY: Simon & Schuster, Inc.

United States Department of Defense. (2012, October). Retrieved from http://www.defense.gov

United States Department of Veteran Affairs. (2012, October). Retrieved from http://www.va.gov

CHAPTER 2

Voices
Understanding the Military Culture as a Context for Delivering Hospice Care: A Practical Application

Deborah Grassman

If a patient maintains his identity as a veteran, the military culture will probably form a significant context in which to provide hospice services. The following story reflects this contextual significance.

> They had been strangers until fate found them as patients in the same room on a VA hospice unit. Luke was a quiet, gentle man. He was paralyzed by a spinal cord compression caused by prostate cancer. He was down to 100 pounds, and his body was contorted like a pretzel. He was also blind from glaucoma. Yet, he emanated serenity. He had a wonderful sense of humor and a youthful giggle that invited everyone into light-heartedness.

> Luke also emanated gratitude. He was grateful to be alive, grateful to receive care, grateful even to be dying because he knew he would soon be home with "my Lord." An elder in his church, Luke was well-known and well-loved in the town's African-American community. Now that he could no longer go to church, his family brought church to him: hymns, communion, scripture, and prayer. When none of his family was around, staff members would play recordings of the Bible or of Mahalia Jackson singing gospel songs.

> There was a genuine holiness in Luke; whenever he spoke, everyone in his presence felt this. Everyone, that is, except his roommate.

Arthur was a gruff ex-Marine Corps sergeant. He admitted to being in pain, but usually refused medication. Instead, he paced. The effects of frostbite from inadequate footgear in the cold regions of Korea had caused some painful nerve damage to his feet; nevertheless, he was grateful that he had not had an amputation the way some of his comrades had.

As Luke had brought everyone into his serenity, Arthur brought everyone into his misery. He was a surly man with little tolerance for anyone's ways except his own. Divorced four times, he claimed all his wives had been "stupid." He was estranged from his children, but his 41-year-old son, Frank, began to visit him. Not having seen his father for 30 years, Frank wanted one last chance to know his father. Arthur frequently snarled and cursed at Frank, yet Frank remained undaunted and stayed faithfully at his father's side.

As a hospice and palliative care nurse practitioner, I made an effort to reach Arthur. "You seem so angry," I said. "It worries me to see how you're pushing everyone away from you."

He shrugged. "They're all morons, that's all," he said contemptuously.

"Is it possible," I asked lightly, "that you're the one being moronic at the moment?"

He scowled, but he didn't push me away.

"You really want everything to go your way," I continued. "Anyone who has other ideas is wrong."

"Yeah," he grunted. "You gotta problem with that?"

"That was important in the military. It worked well then. You were a sergeant and you needed your men to do what you told them to do, but I don't know about now. You might be facing the end of your life in the next several months," I said soberly. "Everything's changing. You might want to think about doing things a little differently now so you can get ready to have a peaceful death, a death without fighting."

Arthur didn't say anything, but I could see him mulling it over. "Maybe…" he said grudgingly and then quickly changed the topic. Motioning toward Luke's bed, he asked to have his room changed. When asked why, he described a racial incident in the Marine Corps in which he had been reprimanded when a subordinate "played the race card against me." We talked about how this incident had intensified his racism. He said he had little use for a blind, paralyzed black man.

I had to resist the urge to move Arthur. It would easily resolve the problem, but it would avoid an opportunity for his making needed inward changes.

"I'll ask Luke and see what he says," I replied. Arthur was used to calling the shots, but I wanted him to know that Luke had a voice in this too. I did not want Arthur's prejudice to affect Luke, but also knew Luke could be a healing influence on Arthur.

I spoke with Luke. He was not fazed by Arthur's mean-spirited assaults. Used to bigotry all his life, Luke shrugged off Arthur's ill temper and laughed with understanding at the proposed room change. Although Arthur did not like it, I decided not to move him to another room.

Over the ensuing weeks, Luke's aura of serenity slowly infiltrated Arthur's side of the room. Arthur complained less about having Luke as a roommate. Gradually, Arthur started seeking the peace he saw in Luke. In the middle of a lonely night, Arthur called to Luke. "You awake, Luke?"

"Yep."

"How about a prayer?"

Luke prayed, and Arthur seemed to surrender some of his anger and bitterness. The stoic wall that had shielded his tender, vulnerable feelings was slowly crumbling. Arthur became more mellow with fewer outbursts of temper.

Luke and Arthur began sharing other things. When Luke's family brought communion, Arthur had communion too. When Arthur went home on the weekends, he would bring back food to share with Luke. Frank talked to the staff about making breakfast for his father in the kitchen on the hospice unit; Arthur asked him to make enough for Luke. When Frank fixed breakfast the next week, Arthur invited the other eight patients on the unit. Mahalia Jackson and the smell of bacon called everyone within hearing and smelling distance to satisfying repast.

The friendship between Luke and Arthur deepened over their weeks together. Possibly for the first time, Arthur was caring about someone other than himself. When Luke needed something, Arthur was there to get it. Conversation drifted between their beds at all hours. A synchrony emerged as though they were still soldiers bonded in the same trench.

One morning as the sun was rising, Luke called out, "You awake, Art?"

"Yeah. What do you need, Luke?"

When Luke didn't respond, Arthur sat up so he could see him more clearly. Luke lay there with his hand outstretched toward Arthur. "I'm dying, Art. The Lord is here for me."

"I'll get someone," Arthur said in a panic. Hurrying from the room, he returned with the housekeeper, Margurite. Luke smiled as the three joined hands. Arthur asked Margurite to pray. When they opened their eyes after the prayer, Luke had died.

Arthur was heartbroken. He beckoned to me as I came down the hallway.

"Luke died, Deborah. I can't believe it. He died." He told and retold their last moments together as if to convince himself of the reality. I put my hand on Arthur's shoulder and said nothing. After a while, he spoke again but he wasn't speaking to me or to anyone in particular. "Tell Luke I'll be joining him soon."

Arthur was given time alone with Luke, but at last it was time to prepare Luke's body for the morgue. Arthur's fierce Marine loyalty would not allow him to leave the room.

"I'm staying right here with him. I'm not going to abandon him now." The room was a foxhole from which these two had faced death together. Luke had carried Arthur through its fire. Now, it was Arthur's turn.

Arthur lingered at the doorway, watching as Luke's body was placed on a morgue cart and an American flag quilt was reverently draped over his body. As Luke's body was transported down the hallway, Arthur raised his hand into a stiff salute. "There goes my best friend," he said, tears streaming down his face. "Who would have ever thought..." he added, his voice trailing off.

Deborah Grassman, ARNP, is a nurse practitioner. Her career at Bay Pines VA in St. Petersburg, FL, lasted for nearly 30 years, where she was the director of the hospice program. She recently retired from the VA and now provides education and consultation throughout the country. Ms. Grassman is the author of Peace at Last: Stories of Hope and Healing for Veterans and Their Families *(Vandamere Press, 2009) and* The Hero Within: Redeeming the Destiny We Were Born to Fulfill *(Vandamere Press, 2012).*

CHAPTER 3

The Military Mindset

James Hallenbeck

> *As we express our gratitude, we must never*
> *forget that the highest appreciation is*
> *not to utter words, but to live by them.*
> ~John Fitzgerald Kennedy

The final chapters of our lives are best understood in the contexts of the stories that precede them. This is as true for veterans as for anyone else. For some veterans their military service represents a core aspect of their identity, a source of great pride. For others, time in military service was but a brief interlude in their life stories. As we explore the important topic of care for veterans at the end of life, we must be mindful of the fact that each veteran lives and carries his or her own story. This chapter will discuss common challenges veterans face toward the end of life and opportunities for clinicians to help veterans and their families meet these challenges. Our collective charge is to help each individual veteran complete his or her final chapter as well as possible, consistent with that veteran's life story. For they have served us. It is an honor for us in turn to serve and to care for them.

For most veterans needing end-of-life care, their time in the service happened many years before, often decades in the past. Veterans vary greatly in the relative importance they attribute to their veteran status. For some veterans military service was a life-long career. Some veterans remain very active in veteran-related activities, such as membership in veteran service organizations like the American Legion or Veterans of Foreign Wars. For some, their sense of identity and their social life is heavily defined by their veteran status. For others, military service was a short-term commitment of relatively minor importance.

Military service, thus, may have had a major or minor impact on individual veterans' lives following their service. This impact may have been extremely positive, helping shape core values, giving rise to discipline, career development opportunities, and social contacts; or it may have been quite negative, as a result of physical or psychological trauma. Some veterans will be very anxious to share their experiences as veterans, as such experiences are central to their being. Other veterans will be quite hesitant, even averse, to discussing their time in the service and the impact of the service on the rest of their lives. In caring for veterans and trying to support them, it is important to respect the great differences in how veterans view and deal with their own veteran status.

MILITARY CULTURE

"Were you in the service?" If there was one critical question we would hope hospice workers would ask of adults coming onto hospice it would be this. If the answer is "Yes," then further exploration of what this means for the individual is a natural next step. But what exactly is "the service?"

Military culture embraces common elements of service, discipline, and mission. In times of war and conflict, service may have involved combat with all that entails: violence, death and the fear of death, and at times great heroism. Service always means some degree of sacrifice. In entering the military one must conform to certain standards of conduct and dress that of necessity impinge on personal liberty. Service may have been entered voluntarily, especially in recent years, or involuntarily through the draft. Regardless, common to military service is the admirable notion of individual sacrifice for the greater good.

No culture is a monolith. For individual veterans their experience of military culture differs significantly based on the time of their service, whether or not service was during a time of conflict or peacetime, the branch of the service in which one served, whether one engaged in or was exposed to combat, and one's rank and role in the service. Military culture also exists within the context of a broader American culture. America's view of the role of the military and military service has fluctuated over time. Shifts in views in popular culture have also influenced military culture and the experiences of those who serve.

TABLE 1

Conflict	Dates	Served	Deaths	Wounded	Death/ Wounded Ratio
World War II	1941 - 1945	16,112,556	405,399	670,846	1:1.65
Korean War	1950 - 1953	5,720,000	36,574	103,284	1:2.8
Vietnam War	1964 - 1973	8,744,000	58,220	153,303[a]	1:2.6
Persian Gulf War	1990 - 1991	2,225,000	383	467	1:1.2
Iraq War	2003 - 2011	?	4,409***	31,430**	1:7.3
War in Afghanistan	2001 - Present	?	1,873***	3,162**	1:4.4

Adapted from: Congressional Research Report, 2012.
*Hospitalized patients, ** As of 7/09, *** As of 6/4/12, Military area of conflict only

World War II (1939-1945) "The Greatest Generation"

In contrast to later conflicts, our country's participation in World War II was broadly supported by the American public. Support for the war effort in and out of uniform was a cultural expectation. Sixteen million Americans, men and women, served during World War II. Four hundred thousand Americans died in the service during the war. Servicemen had long deployments, often lasting up to two years.

Most men and women returning from the war came home to a hero's welcome. As is true for all wars, there was a great cost in lives lost and the damage done to survivors, both veterans and their loved ones. The scope of loss related to WWII is perhaps difficult to imagine in today's world. Given the collective trauma of this war, the emphasis in American culture after the war was on "getting back to normal."

Our oldest group of living veterans now comes from the World War II era. Because of their advanced age it is estimated that 740 WWII veterans pass away each day (National Center for Veterans Analysis and Statistics, 2012).

Veterans of this age group are often frail and prone to diseases and disorders of very old age, such as dementia and strokes. Many are dependent upon others for some assistance.

Korean War (1950-1953) "The Forgotten War"

As the slogan suggests, it is all too easy for people to forget about this conflict and its effect on the 5.7 million Americans who served during this era. 36,574 servicemen died during the conflict. Lacking both the broad cultural support of World War II and the controversy of the Vietnam War, Korean War veterans are at risk for feeling neglected regarding their service and sacrifice. Coming up rapidly behind the World War II generation, this group (and older Vietnam-era veterans) by age are more likely to require hospice care based on diseases affecting adults in their 70s and 80s, such as cancer and chronic conditions such as heart failure and chronic obstructive pulmonary disease.

Vietnam War (1964-1973)

Vietnam was a different war. As compared to World War II and the Korean Conflict, the overall mission was less clear, at least to the general populace. For troops in combat it was also less clear who was a friend and who was the enemy. Our troops were a combination of volunteers and draftees. The American people were sharply divided over the war. American culture more broadly was undergoing rapid changes, influenced by a variety of factors including the civil rights movement, the women's liberation movement, and a powerful anti-war movement. Tragically, many service men and women became lost in this sea of change. Regretfully, many protesting the war seemed unable to separate the war from the warrior. In retrospect, it is fair to say that as a nation in many ways we failed to support this generation of servicemen and women, who too often struggled upon return with problems of substance abuse, unemployment, and a newly identified disorder, Posttraumatic Stress Disorder (PTSD).

Persian Gulf War (1990-1991)

Two million Americans served during this relatively brief war; 383 servicemen died during the conflict.

Wars in Afghanistan (2001-present) and Iraq (2003-2011)

While formally distinguished as separate military operations, these two conflicts significantly overlap in time periods, deployments (servicemen and women may have been deployed to Afghanistan or Iraq, or have been deployed to both), the type of conflicts in which troops engaged, and the associated challenges faced. As was true for the Persian Gulf War, our troops were volunteers. The nature of the conflicts, with disproportionately more casualties due to improvised explosive devices (IEDs) and fewer casualties from traditional weaponry resulted in very low death-to-wounded ratios, as reflected in Table 1. Death rates in these conflicts were low, at least relative to those in Vietnam and earlier conflicts. While lower death rates are welcomed, a significant number of the wounded suffered amputations and traumatic brain injuries resulting from blast injuries. 1,448 servicemen and women had some form of amputation (Congressional Research Report, 2012).

Not all wounds are visible. The exact number of veterans suffering from PTSD or depression related to these conflicts is not known.

Veteran Demographics

As the above discussion suggests, each veteran's story is unique. A general understanding of demographic patterns and trends may help clinicians appreciate the circumstances and contexts giving rise to these stories.

As of November 2011, it is estimated that there were 22,234,000 veterans (7% of U.S. population) in the United States, of which 8% were women (National Center for Veterans Analysis and Statistics, 2012; Women Veterans Health Strategic Health Care Group, 2010). 1,711,000 of these were WWII veterans of which it is estimated that 740 die each day. 42% of the veteran population is 65 or older. 78.7% of veterans are white, 11.6% black, 6.0% Hispanic, with Asian/Pacific islanders, American Indians/Alaskan Natives and other groups compromising the remaining 3.7%. In 2011, 8.47 million (38.1%) of all veterans were enrolled for care through the VA and 6,166,000 (27.5%) received some care through the VA during that year. An unpublished study by Hallenbeck and Breckenridge, examining veteran deaths in 2001, demonstrated in that year that of approximately 25 million veterans, 674,000 died; that figure represents a remarkable 28% of total deaths in the US, more than all deaths in the US due to cancer. Of these, 104,234 (15.5%) were enrolled and received some care from the VA, of which only 28,879 (4.3%) died as inpatients in VA facilities, either in VA acute care hospitals or nursing homes. At present it is estimated that approximately 642,000 veterans die each year, of which 21,000 (3.3%) die in VA facilities (Department of Veterans Affairs, 2011). Approximately 30% of these 642,000 veterans will have used some VA resources in the last year of life. Over the past decade the number of veterans dying each year has decreased approximately 5% and fewer veterans are dying as VA inpatients. The large percentage (96.7%) of veterans dying outside a VA institution, some of whom had received prior care through the VA and many of whom did not, highlights the importance of VA and community collaborations.

From this basic demographic information we can distill some key points:

- While veterans currently represent less than 10% of the U.S. population, because of the very large number of WWII and Korean War-era veterans, who are now of advanced age, approximately one in four deaths is that of a veteran.
- Because older-era veterans were overwhelmingly male, of older dying men, more than 50% of those older than 65 are veterans.
- A majority of veterans receive their care outside of the VA system. The majority will die under the direct care of non-VA providers.

Let us consider for a moment some of the implications of the above. An underlying tenet of this book is that veteran status is a relevant factor to consider in the care of a seriously ill or dying patient. Veteran status may or may not be important for the individual patient or family member, but we would argue that assessment of veteran status is important enough that it warrants routine assessment, much like age, gender, or ethnicity.

Exactly why is such assessment important? For the purposes of this section, beyond providing us opportunities for statements of respect and gratitude for services rendered, it should be enough that any factor or variable that is associated with as much as 25% of all deaths and 50% of all older male deaths is worthy of focused, systematic attention.

Clinical needs of veterans

Clinically, veteran needs and preferences at the end of life are more similar than not to those of non-veterans (Steinhauser et al., 2000). Most veterans die of the same spectrum of diseases that non-veterans do; with these come a similar range of symptom management challenges. Some veterans will carry with them physical disabilities associated with their time in service that contribute to their net symptom burden. For example, veterans exposed to artillery blasts may suffer deafness or ringing in the ears. Old war wounds may have given rise to chronic pains that underlay pain syndromes of more recent onset. Some veterans may die from disease known to be associated with some military exposure. For example, Navy or shipyard workers exposed to asbestos may develop lung cancer possibly associated with that exposure. While such service-associated illnesses may not differ significantly in their clinical presentation, the veteran's understanding of the illness may differ significantly, if it is believed to be associated with time in the service.

Possible associations between illnesses and service need not be as straightforward as asbestos exposure or war wounds. Veterans may perceive less obvious connections. For example, veterans may have started smoking or drinking in the service and associate later disease with these behaviors and service time. Clinically, the issue is not so much whether the service was to blame for whatever happened, but more one of getting a clearer picture of how the individual and his or her family understands the illness in the context, if any, of military service. Attribution in some way to military service may give rise to anger or increased symptomatology, if the association is negatively framed in terms of regret, injustice, or blame. On the other hand, coping can be enhanced and symptomatology reduced if and when associated illness is understood in a positive context of service, duty, and honor.

While physical symptomatology among veterans is quite similar to that of non-veterans, veterans may experience special challenges psychologically, socially, and spiritually in approaching the ends of their lives. While a detailed review of these challenges is beyond the scope of this chapter, we can briefly highlight some more common issues about which to be aware.

For many veterans their most direct exposure to death and dying may have occurred during time in the service. If exposed to combat, death and dying may be consciously or unconsciously linked to the violence of war, triggering difficult and painful memories. Some veterans may present with known PTSD. Others, especially older-era veterans of the Korean War and World War II, may not carry such a formal diagnosis, but may have PTSD-like symptomatology unmasked through the process of dying. The emergence or exacerbation of PTSD-like symptoms may occur, not just because of the threat of impending death, but also because carefully constructed coping mechanisms may unwind through the process of advanced illness. Advanced illness and dying unavoidably entail uncertainty and dependence on others, both of which can be particularly difficult for people with PTSD (Feldman and Periyakoil, 2006; Grassman, 2007).

Veterans vary in the relative importance of their time in military service and how this aspect of their lives is integrated into or segregated from the rest of their social lives. As previously mentioned, for some, involvement in military-related activities, such as veteran service groups, is a critical aspect of their social identity. Recognition of this, statements of appreciation and respect for service, and promotion of continued involvement of support networks, if possible, may significantly bolster quality of life. Conversely, sudden separation or isolation from such support may trigger grief and depression. Some veterans may have decided not to talk about their time in service with family and friends, especially regarding painful or difficult experiences. While family members may have gotten used to the fact that "Dad doesn't talk about what happened in the war," this gap in the individual veteran's and the family's life narratives may come to the fore during the process of dying. As a part of their life reviews preceding death, veterans and their loved ones may struggle to integrate difficult, often unspoken chapters into their life stories. Hospice workers as empathetic listeners may play an important role in helping veterans and their families better integrate these stories.

Spiritual issues may arise for anybody facing mortality. Combat veterans may struggle to reconcile the trauma of war with personal beliefs and values. Veterans may try to reconcile beliefs, for example, in the sanctity of life with military values, stressing mission and national defense. If directly involved in activities that might violate some moral or ethical code, such as the taking of life, even where such action might be necessary or required within a military role, moral distress or injury may occur (Litz et al., 2009). Sensitivity to the possibility of such distress in veterans and attention to it, when it arises, is critical in the provision of good spiritual care.

Here are some helpful ways to support veterans:
- Ask people if they were in the service and if so, which branch.
- Thank veterans for their service.
- Express interest in their experiences and invite them to share their stories.
- Avoid stereotyping by service or period of service. Individual veterans likely had very different experiences in the service.

THE ROLE OF THE DEPARTMENT OF VETERANS AFFAIRS (VA)

A common misconception is that all care provided to veterans is provided by the VA. Clearly, this is not the case, particularly as relates to end-of-life care. The VA is more likely to provide care to certain subsets of the veteran population; those with "service-connected disabilities" (a formal VA determination of a disability linked in some way to time spent in military service), or those of lower socioeconomic status, such as homeless veterans.

TABLE 2

Characteristics of Veterans Enrolled in VA at the Time of Death	
Age	• 86.8% are 65 years or older • Average age at death is mid-70s and rising
Gender	• 97.5% male • Women smaller part of the military during World War II, Korean and Vietnam conflicts
Marital Status	• 41% married • 59% divorced or separated, widowed, or never married
Race	• 78% Caucasian • 17% African American • < 5% other racial backgrounds
Diagnosis	• 55% of VA inpatient deaths overall have a cancer diagnosis • 70% of VA inpatient deaths in hospice bed sections have a cancer diagnosis
Hospice Coverage	• Medicare is the primary payer for hospice care nationally • 78.5% Veterans enrolled in VA at time of death also enrolled in Medicare • 80% of enrolled Veterans over 65 also enrolled in Medicare

From 2011 Hospice and Palliative Care Report, Office of Geriatrics and Extended Care.

Why is most care for veterans toward the end of life provided outside the VA? The vast majority of veterans over age 65 have Medicare. Of veterans enrolled in the VA, 86.5% are 65 or older at the time of death; 78.5% of all decedents are also enrolled in Medicare at the time of death. Many veterans live at some distance from their local VA facility and with increasing frailty many may find it more convenient to receive care closer to home. Dual eligibility between VA and Medicare makes this possible for many. If enrolled, many veterans living at a distance may choose to receive certain services from the VA, while using local resources for other healthcare needs. Like most Americans, most veterans would likely prefer to die at home.

That this is the case has important implications. Attending to the end-of-life needs of veterans cannot be the sole responsibility of the Department of Veterans Affairs; clearly, this will require a community effort. That many veterans will receive care through the VA and non-VA agencies suggests both opportunities and challenges. The great opportunity is for us to work together, VA and non-VA partners, utilizing our particular strengths toward a common purpose of serving the veteran. On the flip side, the equally great challenge is to try to ensure that veterans do not fall through the cracks of different healthcare systems. In many cases the problem is as simple as misunderstanding or ignorance of what might be available to help veterans. Even where individuals and agencies share a common commitment to improving care for veterans, the complexities of our healthcare systems are such that it is far too easy to not know what services are available and how best to access them.

What services are available through the VA?

The Department of Veterans Affairs is a large government agency with multiple functions. Total government appropriations for 2011 exceeded $125 billion dollars (National Center for Veterans Analysis and Statistics, 2012). One of these functions is the direct provision of benefits to veterans and their families. In fact, this is the primary function of one branch of the Department, the Veterans Benefit Administration (VBA). The other branch, the Veterans Health Administration (VHA), is involved in the direction provision of healthcare for enrolled veterans, much like a health maintenance organization (HMO). Of particular interest to hospice workers, the VBA oversees burial and memorial benefits. Some families may also be eligible for survivor benefits, especially for veterans dying of illnesses related to their service-connected disabilities.

At present the VHA operates 152 hospitals across the country and over 800 associated outpatient clinics, called Community Based Outpatient Clinics (CBOCs). These hospitals and clinics provide a wide array of medical and mental health services, similar to large HMOs. Beyond this, the VA specializes in the delivery of certain services not commonly available in the private sector, such as spinal cord injury care, blind rehabilitation, rehabilitative care for homeless veterans, and non-institutional home care, such as a Home-Based Primary Care (HBPC) program, in which VA clinicians provide care directly to homebound patients. As discussed further in a later chapter the VA also directly provides hospice and palliative care services to enrolled veterans.

Is the VA a form of health insurance?

This is a complicated topic, prone to misunderstanding. While the VA does "cover" healthcare expenses for certain enrolled veterans in certain circumstances (beyond the scope of this review), in most cases it is best to think of VA hospitals and associated clinics as healthcare providers, charged with providing care for patients enrolled with particular VA hospitals and associated clinics. Understanding this is important because community hospices sometimes contact VA facilities, asking for payment for a service after-the-fact or asking for hospice coverage for a veteran who is not enrolled with a VA facility. The VA lacks the authority to pay for such services for veterans not enrolled for care. Hospice care in the community, when it is authorized, must be approved in advance administratively and clinically by a VA physician.

VA facilities are required to either provide or purchase hospice services for enrolled veterans meeting VA eligibility standards. As one might expect, there are numerous details regarding processes and procedures for doing this. Community hospice workers are referred to their local VA facility hospice and palliative care clinical and programmatic representatives for such details. Below are listed some general points to bear in mind if contacting or working with a VA facility regarding a veteran and hospice care:

- VA facilities are restricted to providing support for enrolled veterans only. If a veteran is not enrolled, in many cases this can be done rather quickly, if proper paperwork is available (discharge papers), but it really helps to think ahead if anticipating a need for a currently unenrolled veteran (for enrollment information see https://www.1010ez.med.va.gov/).
- Veterans need to be enrolled at a particular VA facility. Most commonly, this is the facility responsible for veterans within a particular geographic catchment area. However, if an enrolled veteran has recently moved, he or she may be enrolled at a different facility. Check with the veteran as to which VA facility he or she is enrolled. Inquiries are generally best started with that facility.
- Most, but not all, enrolled veterans will have a VA primary care provider responsible for that veteran's overall care. Ask the veteran if he or she has such a provider and ask for the provider's name. Connecting with this provider, if possible, is the best way to coordinate care.

- If working to obtain hospice services for an enrolled veteran through the VA, the VA assumes that they will either provide such services (usually through VA facility inpatient hospice programs) or a VA provider will order such services be provided through a community agency. For dually eligible veterans (most commonly VA and Medicare) who meet VA criteria for hospice care it is the veteran's choice as to whether the VA pays for the care or the veteran elects the Medicare Hospice Benefit. Regardless, if working through the VA, a VA physician must place an order for admission to hospice. What does not work is for a non-VA provider or agency to determine that a veteran qualifies for hospice and then calls a VA facility, expecting authorization or payment for care by a community agency with no order in advance by a VA physician. In this regard the VA does not function like an insurance agency. Thus, if anticipating a need for VA support of a veteran in a community hospice program, it is critical to ensure that veteran is enrolled and connected to a VA provider, who can coordinate care.
- When caring for a veteran referred for hospice care by a VA physician, the physician may or may not elect to serve as attending of record for the veteran. Where a physician declines to be attending of record or is unable to so serve (some VA physicians may not have a state license in the state of the hospice agency), alternative arrangements for an attending should be sought.
- Community hospice agencies already caring for a veteran through a non-VA funding source, most commonly Medicare, may still request assistance from a VA facility for an enrolled veteran. Usually, this occurs when inpatient hospice care is desired. VA facilities vary in their procedures and availability of inpatient hospice beds. Agencies should ask to speak to VA facility hospice or palliative care coordinators to discuss details.

James Hallenbeck, MD, is an associate professor of medicine at Stanford University in the Division of General Medical Disciplines. He is Associate Chief of Staff for Extended Care and director of Palliative Care Services at VA Palo Alto Health Care System. He is board certified in Internal Medicine and Hospice and Palliative Medicine. He was the project chair for a national Veterans Affairs taskforce (TAPC) which worked to expand and improve palliative care throughout the VA. He is the hub-site director for a fellowship program in palliative care offered by the VA at six training sites across the country, called the Interprofessional Palliative Care Fellowship Program. Dr. Hallenbeck's academic interests in the area of palliative care have included physician education, non-pain symptom management, and cultural aspects of end-of-life care. He is the author of the book Palliative Care Perspectives *(Oxford University Press, 2003).*

REFERENCES

Congressional Research Report, *American War and Military Operations Casualties.* (Updated 2010, February 26). Retrieved from http://www.fas.org/sgp/crs/natsec/RL32492.pdf.

Department of Veterans Affairs, Patient Care Services. (2011). *Department of Veterans Affairs Hospice and Palliative Care 2011 Annual Report.* Washington, DC: Author.

Feldman, D.B., & Periyakoil, V.S. (2006). Posttraumatic stress disorder at the end of life. *Journal of Palliative Medicine, 9*(1), 213-8.

Grassman, D. (2007). Wounded warriors: Their last battle. *Home Health Nurse, 25*(5), 299-304.

Hallenbeck, J., & Breckenridge, J. (2001). *Veteran Deaths in VA.* Unpublished Manuscript.

Litz, B.T., Stein, N., Delaney, E., Lebowitz, L., Nash, W.P., Silva, C., & Maguen, S. (2009). Moral injury and moral repair in war veterans: A preliminary model and intervention strategy. *Clinical Psychology Review, 29*(8), 695-706.

National Center for Veterans Analysis and Statistics. (2012). *VA Benefits and Healthcare Utilization.* Washington, DC: Department of Veterans Affairs.

Steinhauser, K.E., Christakis, N.A., Clipp, A.C., McNeilly, M., McIntyre, L., & Tulsky, J.A. (2000). Factors considered important at the end of life by patients, family, physicians, and other care providers. *JAMA, 284*(19), 2476-82.

Women Veterans Health Strategic Health Care Group, Veterans Health Administration. (2010). *Sourcebook: Women Veterans in the Veterans Health Administration, Vol. 1.* Washington, DC: Author.

CHAPTER 4

Voices
Why Didn't Anyone Ever Ask?

David Abrams

In 2006 I attended a workshop for clinicians in end-of-life care. At the start of the workshop the presenters asked any veterans present to raise their hands. I raised mine, as did two or three others. They then thanked us for our service and went on with the workshop agenda. I was puzzled and bothered over why I was being thanked. I had known the workshop instructors personally and professionally for several years. They were knowledgeable, experienced, and well-meaning professional caregivers. Even five years after 9/11, our national self-consciousness over acknowledging veterans and first responders was at a high point. Yet I was embarrassed because over 40 years had passed since I left the military, and I certainly did not feel like a hero; in 2006, I was thinking of Iraq and Afghanistan veterans. This "thank you" struck me as formulaic, inorganic, and more of a way to help the instructors present to feel better. If they want to really thank us for our service, I thought, there must be better ways to do it.

In the years since this event, it has occurred to me that healthcare clinicians could maintain an effective advocacy for veterans by virtue of their strategic spot on the diagnostic team. Veterans often have odd medical complications that the veteran him or herself might not be able to trace back to a cause, or there may be underlying pathologies or conditions that may be hidden to the veteran. A clinician who is aware that the patient is a veteran can play a key role in helping to crack a mysterious medical condition. This would be a wonderful way to honor our veterans, much more meaningful and significant than just lapel pins and thank yous.

My own bizarre and dangerous experience with the medical system that started in 2000, in what turned out to be a service-connected disability, may help serve as an example. A four-and-one-half year odyssey could have been cut to perhaps six months if any clinician had just asked me if I was a veteran. That simple question could have led to an early diagnosis of my illness, saving time, anguish, and money. It is speculative (but not unreasonably so) to expect a better outcome if any one of a variety of clinicians had made the thought progression: "old guy—veteran—Vietnam veteran...Agent Orange."

I had served in South Vietnam in 1962. Although that was very early in U.S. involvement, the Air Force began spraying the country with various toxins in 1961. I was discharged in 1964 and went about building a life as a civilian. For the next 34 years I led a relatively normal life in terms of health and wellness. In November 1998, I began to lose feeling in my feet, and by the following February a numbness had spread to my ankles. By May 1999, the numbness was joined by pain. I felt as if I was walking on my bones, with no padding, and my feet hurt as if they were stuck in an electrical outlet. Most diabetics understand that this pain is neuropathic and know how intense it can be.

At this point I needed to get some understanding of what was going on, and so began 56 months of testing, perhaps some mismanagement, and a failure of understanding of pain issues. And this was all conducted by the most wonderful, well-meaning, committed group of physicians one might find. Unfortunately, well-meaning can be dangerous.

My primary care physician immediately tested me for diabetes, but the tests were all negative. For the pain we tried aspirin, ibuprofen, heat, ice, water massage, and hand massage. A podiatrist performed an ultrasound on my legs, found some blockages, and suggested a vascular workup. Taking that suggestion I transferred to an academic hospital, where a vascular surgeon ordered ultrasounds of the carotid artery and aorta, four MRIs, a barium swallow, and glucose tolerance tests. He rejected foot and vascular problems as a cause of the neuropathy and gave me an orthotic device. He also suggested a neurological workup, so I went to a neurologist at a Parkinson's institute where I had some manometry testing. No apparent reason for the neuropathy was evident.

Complaining about the severe neuropathic pain, I was prescribed Amytriptiline, but was unable to tolerate it; I found myself constantly drowsy, even to the point of falling asleep at my desk. Desperate for effective pain control, I began acupuncture and alternative treatments, including diet modification such as substituting organic foods for non-organic, and nutritional supplements. The acupuncture noticeably reduced the pain as long as I could get treatments every three days, and the acupuncturist added Chinese herbs and electric current.

I concomitantly had dental surgery and my dentist prescribed Percoset for postoperative pain. Surprise! The neuropathic pain disappeared immediately and completely and I thought I had a miracle in hand. But neither my primary care physician nor my neurologist would prescribe Percoset, other than a few low doses at a time. My neurologist prescribed Neurontin for the pain.

A referral to a well-known clinic for more neural examinations resulted in electromyogram and nerve conduction tests. We changed my cholesterol medication from a statin to a non-statin. In response to increasing pain, the neurologist tripled the Neurontin dosage to 900 mg, 3 times a day. Then things got really interesting.

In 2001 I relocated my office. I was unable to get my new location organized; I kept misplacing files and I lost my bathroom keys twice. Daily tasks and movements dulled. When leaving my house in the morning I would have to return three or four times to get all the things I needed for the day. One time I put something in the trunk of my car, then pulled out of the driveway without closing the trunk. I once came out of the bathroom in my house with my fly open, and I even did that in public. I had two near misses while changing lanes in my car, both of which were my fault. I was a premium status flyer with over 50,000 miles a year. But when a flight I was on got cancelled, I could not understand what I had to do, even when it was explained to me. All this occurred in one month.

The next month, I lost an airline ticket; it turned out that I had thrown it away. One very disturbing incident occurred when I received $500 in cash to deposit to my bank account. I put it in my wallet, then promptly forgot about it. I discovered the $500 six days later and had trouble remembering why it was in my wallet.

At the end of the summer of 2001 I stepped off a curb in Washington, DC, and right into oncoming traffic. A taxi's brakes screeched as its bumper stopped inches from my leg. I sat down on the curb; for a few minutes, I thought I would throw up. The final straw came when my wife confronted me with her observation of my lost mental acuity and behavioral issues. She said for the past few weeks I had been challenging her on everything she said. I argued with her (of course), but then that weekend I almost caused another accident by cutting off a car near my home. It was a very close call that was only prevented by the other driver's alertness.

I called my doctor to discuss the adverse reaction to the increased Neurontin. He said that maybe I was under stress and was not concentrating when I stepped into traffic. I became infuriated. I screamed into the phone,

"I was born and raised in New York City and lived there for 33 years. It is biologically and organically impossible for a New Yorker to step off a curb into traffic. You're blaming me, the patient for this? You go f**k yourself, you're fired." I thought it only fair that this extreme behavioral aberration should be directed against the doctor who prescribed the drug. I had taken my last dose of Neurontin.

I continued taking Percoset which was the only effective treatment for my pain, getting it wherever I could. I also tried LED devices for pain relief, to no effect. A well-known pain expert I knew encouraged me to stop self-treating and helped me get to an academic hospital with a pain center. The pain specialists first prescribed Trileptal, which I was unable to tolerate. They then prescribed Fentanyl, Percoset for breakthrough pain and, finally, Methadone. I felt like I had stepped from a black bog into Shangri-la. The pain relief was complete and I had no side effects other than some minor energy issues, which adjusted themselves. By the end of the year, and for the first time in 56 months, my pain was under control. It has been under control since then with a dose of 5 mg of Methadone 2-3 times per day, essentially the same dosage at which I started.

With my pain under control I could at last regain control of my life. However, the cause of the neuropathy was still unknown and we did not seem to be getting any closer. It was clear that each clinician could only react within the context of his or her specialty. I needed someone who could design and manage a rational, unified approach to gaining an understanding of the pathologies, someone who was motivated to solve the medical mystery engulfing my body. Instead, each doctor I saw conducted whatever tests he trusted and then referred me to a colleague. Each referral sounded to me like another way of giving up. So the search for the cause of the neuropathy was effectively over, but I didn't care as long as the pain was under control.

One day while I was in DC I was near the Vietnam Veterans Memorial and stopped at the table run by the Vietnam Veterans of America. We started talking about the neuropathy and the guy asked me if I served in Vietnam. When I told him I did, he gave me a brochure and said, "Man, you need to look at the Agent Orange part of our website." That night I did and I was stunned. Every single symptom, pain issue, and emotion that I felt was there; there was nothing secret, magical, or mysterious about it. The VA had listed 11 diseases as presumptively caused by Agent Orange, and non-diabetic neuropathy was one of them. Thousands of veterans had experienced the same thing as me. I was no longer alone.

But what about the doctors I had seen? There were so many of them. Forget asking about Vietnam; not one single doctor had even asked me if I'd been in the military. If one doctor had expressed a scientist's interest in the mystery of my illness, perhaps that may have encouraged a forensic approach. But they had a convenient word for it: "idiopathic" or no apparent cause, and that was the answer, even though by definition it is not an answer. Think what it would have meant for my diagnosis if just one doctor had asked, "Are you a veteran?" and followed that line of inquiry for a while. How much shorter and less costly would the arc of care had been?

In the first Gulf War our troops were breathing burning oil. Soon they will be approaching two decades removed from that war; what a convenient time for lung conditions to manifest themselves. Iraq and Afghanistan have brought us only to the beginnings of learning about traumatic brain injury, but it may again be decades before symptoms manifest. Women are challenging the traditional notion of combat injuries, and what do we know about how those might affect women's health issues? Physicians must begin to look outside their diagnostic toolbox when answers to clinical problems are not apparent.

How might this work down the line? It seems to me a good deal of it is about awareness. If you are treating a patient of a certain age and if he or she is presenting strange symptoms (or normal symptoms that do not fit the current context), inquire into veteran status. Be aware that veterans can have odd medical complications that they cannot trace back in a lineal manner. Clinicians such as nurses, physician assistants, nurse practitioners, and even social workers, are in an excellent position to influence the view the physician sees.

Many veterans just want to get back to a normal life. But for the ill veteran, who is reminded every day of that service, how can you honor him or her more than by knowing how to adequately care for them by understanding the underlying cause of their illness? This, it seems to me, would be a meaningful way to say thank you to our veterans and a sincere way to honor them.

David Abrams *was the senior operations officer and CEO of Hospice Foundation of America (HFA) from 1990 through 2008, a national charity that educates in end-of-life issues. Now retired, he serves on the board of HFA. As CEO he was responsible for overall administrative, business development, marketing, fundraising, and program responsibilities. Prior to joining Hospice Foundation of America Abrams was a regional manager for a nationwide savings bank, a legislative analyst in the Florida Senate, and worked in the fire protection industry. He served four years in the U.S. Marine Corps. Abrams currently serves as a board member of the Health and Medical Research Charities of America Federation and as a mentor on the Broward County Veteran's Court. He has served on the National Community AIDS Partnership and was a director of the Miami-Dade Task Force for Battered Women.*

CHAPTER 5

Generational Cohorts: A Military Perspective

Kenneth J. Doka

I n a 1986 Presidential Address to the American Sociological Association, Matilda White Riley noted the often-neglected study of age cohorts. Riley reiterated that age cohorts, or generations, were often overlooked in sociology. To Riley, generational cohorts were a significant source of diversity; each cohort or generation was shaped by unique social, historical, and demographic factors that influenced their attitudes, values, and behaviors. As such they shaped the ways that a generation responded to crises such as life-limiting illness and end-of-life care as well as the way members of a cohort might interact with counselors and health professionals.

This may be particularly true with military cohorts. Here two factors converge. First are the generational differences that exist between veterans of different wars. Regardless of whether there was military service, each generation shared distinct and differentiating experiences. There are differences between the GI Generation shaped in the forge of the Depression and World War II and those of the Baby Boomers primarily born after World War II. Second, each cohort of veterans also was affected by their shared combat experiences. Those who fought in World War II had very different experiences than the veterans of the wars in Korea and Vietnam. In understanding the importance of generational cohorts, we need not lose the individual. As with any source of diversity, it important to remember what is called the *ecological fallacy*; that is, that generalizations that hold for a group may not necessarily apply to all members of that group.

The study of cohorts, though, reinforces an important point; systems of care need to be reassessed and reinvented as each new cohort ages. Such reimagining involves intergenerational considerations, such as Baby Boomers managing care of Traditional Generation parents. It is also important to recognize that cohorts are socially constructed; thus different writers may use somewhat different years or terms to define cohort. In this chapter we primarily follow the listings offered by Strauss and Howe (1991).

THE VETERAN EXPERIENCE

There is a proverb that states: *Every person is like all other persons, some other persons, no other person.* Certainly all humans share basic characteristics and needs. And as noted earlier, we can never lose sight of the uniqueness of every individual. Yet individuals who share a culture, a lifestyle, a social class, spirituality, or experience (among other factors) do share certain commonalities.

Military culture often values hierarchy, interdependence, respect for authority, heroic sacrifice, patriotism, and risk-taking. Stoicism is prized. These values may not mesh well with end-of-life care as individuals may be forced into dependency and encouraged to make autonomous choices. Moreover, the shared experiences of military veterans in combat may result in difficult memories and even the re-emergence of earlier symptoms of Posttraumatic Stress Disorder (PTSD) at the end of life. These experiential components may clash with the practices often employed in end-of-life care that affirm open emotionality and grieving, as well as those that encourage reminiscence and life review.

While these elements of military culture are common to most veterans, cohorts also matter. Often the GI Generation (born between 1901-1924) and the Silent Generation (born between 1925-1942) are now grouped together as the Traditional Generation as they share common experiences of later life; many of their formative experiences were not radically different, such as growing up in intact homes, utilizing savings accounts, and experiencing radio and newspaper as major informational sources. As a group, the members of the Traditional Generation often accept the fact that life is unfair, and may be more accepting of their fate. Traditionalists, after all, grew up at a time when medical treatments were limited. They lived in an era prior to penicillin and other antibiotics, and some remember the many epidemics such as the Flu Pandemic. They also lived through the demographic transition; many saw parents or siblings die from diseases easily cured now. Children died from polio or whooping cough, and heart attacks were fatal. Therefore, some may be fatalistic and view medications and hospitals with suspicion. Yet they were a group that accepted authority. Raised in the Depression and war years, they looked to the government for assistance. Since they learned to follow orders, they remain generally adherent, often seeking a doctor's advice for anything health-related and rarely questioning physicians.

While end-of-life preparation meant wills and other estate planning, Traditionalists will now accept the need for healthcare proxies and advance directives. With increasing dependence they may have conflicts with Baby Boomer caregivers on "downsizing." Living through a depression may have made them wary of the perceived wastefulness of their Boomer children as their offspring attempt to toss out "clutter." Because they struggled to achieve prosperity and regard savings accounts and homes as prized symbols of achievement and security, Traditionalists may seriously struggle with difficult decisions regarding savings and assets when considering eligibility for government programs.

Traditionalists tend to be quiet about emotions and feelings and are generally resistant to therapy, as they defined therapy as being for persons who were "crazy." They are, though, the first generation to embrace widow/widower and other grief support groups, perhaps as a reflection of their "can-do" orientation, which values strength in the face of difficulty.

There are distinct ethnic differences among Traditionalists. African Americans in these generations experienced harsh discrimination and prejudice, themes that may emerge in life review. Many persons may have a pride of survivorship, a sense that they have lived through a range of life experiences both as individuals and as a race, from harsh segregation to the election of an African-American president. African-American Traditionalists remember the Tuskegee Syphilis Study, which caused distrust of medical professionals. Many also have strong spiritual beliefs such as a strong trust in the miraculous action of God and the strong value placed on life and the pride of survivorship. These beliefs, combined with a general mistrust of medical authority, may lead to reluctance to consider palliative care.

The military experiences of these two "traditional" generations, though, are quite different. The GI Generation fought in World War II, a war of shared sacrifice. While the experiences of the GIs were often difficult, they perceived national support. As they liberated countries from brutal Axis occupiers, they were greeted by delirious populations. They returned to victory parades that honored them for their service. The Servicemen's Readjustment Act of 1944 (commonly known as the G.I. Bill), passed by a grateful nation, opened up opportunities such as higher education and home ownership.

While the Silent Generation, the generation now often seen in end-of-life care, shared many of the cohort experiences of the GI experience, their combat experiences were very different. The Silent Generation veterans fought, for the most part, in the Korean War. This war was one of the first armed conflicts of the Cold War as the communist North Korea invaded the South. It was a difficult conflict. Cold was as much an enemy as the communists. For those on the front, there was often tedium and isolation; much of the fighting was at night. There was the frustration expressed by General Douglas MacArthur that political considerations to localize the war meant that the US was not using the full force of their offensive capabilities. For three years, American and United Nation armies battled North Korean and intervening Chinese armies until both sides accepted an armistice and cold peace that essentially confirmed the pre-war status quo. Yet nearly half of the American casualties occurred after the peace talks commenced.

These veterans returned to a war-weary population largely content to ignore the sacrifices made. The war did not have a glorious conclusion, so it was quickly forgotten, relegated to the history books. There were few parades to honor veterans. Moreover, veterans returned to the US during a recession, finding limited opportunities for employment.

The Baby Boomer Generation, born between 1943 and 1960, also had very different experiences. Births deferred by the Depression and World War II soared as servicemen began to return home from that war. The sheer size of the Boom, now 73 million, meant that Baby Boomers faced competition and crowds at every stage of life. They were the first generation influenced by television. Boomers were a generation of worsening trends as divorce and delinquency rates rose. Their experience of government was shaped by Watergate and Vietnam, a far different outlook than their parents' experiences of the New Deal and a unified war effort.

The Boomer Generation is also very diverse both ethnically and spiritually. The 1965 Immigration Act eliminated quotas and allowed migration from countries previously limited or excluded. Spiritual diversity was also evident in the growth of non-Western religions. The Baby Boomer Generation experienced the sexual revolution and was active in the women's and gay rights movements.

Military experience is another source of significant diversity for Boomers. Veterans of this generation primarily saw combat in the Vietnam War, in many ways creating a generational rift that may still persist. This was a war against a shadowy guerrilla army; it was unclear as to who was friend, neutral, or foe. While returning Korean War veterans may have been met with indifference, Vietnam Veterans often encountered hostility, particularly from their peers. Unlike World War II, only a minority of peers actually served in the armed forces. There were other differences as well. Unlike the liberated people of WWII or even the Koreans, few Vietnamese welcomed the Americans. There was no sense of shared purpose and there was ambiguity about goals; both factors eroded morale as did the open and robust organized opposition to the war in the US and Europe.

Boomers changed every social institution they encountered. Boomer values of individuality, personal autonomy, and distrust of authority challenged colleges and workplaces. Boomers are now aging; by 2030, when all Boomers are over 65, 18% of the U.S. population will be 65 or older. It will be interesting to see the ways that Boomers may challenge how we age and die.

Boomers are likely to offer challenges to traditional end-of-life care. Medicine made great strides in the Boomer Generation. Boomers saw the conquest of polio and tremendous advances in all forms of treatment, so they may be reluctant to accept that care may now be palliative and not curative. Moreover, Boomers will expect to be actively involved in determining their medical care rather than simply accepting medical authority. Boomers are heavy consumers of alternative treatments including chiropractors, acupuncture, herbal and natural treatments, and vitamins, and may also be more prone to use non-prescribed drugs. The Boomer Generation was one of the first to widely experiment with recreational drugs.

Boomers value "death with dignity," as well as effective pain management; they were at the forefront of the hospice movement, so that portends well for hospice use as Boomers age. On the other hand, control and options might make hospice more attractive if it offers concurrent care, the option to receive hospice care along with disease-modifying treatments. Wright and Katz (2007), for example, recount a case where a woman opted out of hospice since it did not offer life-extending treatment nor nutritional support, and the patient wanted to survive until her daughter's wedding. In addition, Boomer focus on autonomy and control may lead to some interesting ethical dilemmas. For example, some Boomers have stated in advance directives that if they do not know enough to eat, they do not want to be fed.

As a generation, Boomers grew up with guidance counselors so are not generally averse to therapy, although receptiveness to therapy is mediated by other variables such as class or ethnicity. Boomers too embraced self-help movements, especially as self-help turned from prohibitory to enhancing; that is, from keeping an individual from doing something such as turning to alcohol to helping them cope with and transform their life. Strength-based approaches are often useful as Boomers are independent, accustomed to challenging authority, and often have a strong sense of self-efficacy. Life review can assist Boomers in identifying the ways they responded to earlier challenges. Yet Boomers may very well have issues that arise in counseling. Boomers were the first "Me Generation," often putting their aspirations ahead of others' needs. High divorce rates, more women in the workplace, and higher rates of single-parent families meant that their children were the first latch-key generation. Wanting first to be friends to their children, they were often permissive. Living in a highly competitive world, relationships took a back seat. Thus issues of guilt and regret may arise in counseling.

Clinicians need to be aware of both generational differences in general and the ways that military experience may have interacted with those generational differences in ways that might influence care. There are instruments such as the *Military History Checklist* that can be a useful part of intake assessment. (A copy of the Checklist can be found in the Resource section of this book.) At a very basic level, this may have residual health effects. World War II veterans who fought in the South Pacific may have suffered a variety of tropical diseases such as malaria. Korean War veterans may have experienced extreme cold, suffering from frostbite and hypothermia. Many Vietnam veterans were exposed to Agent Orange and have high rates of testing positive for the Hepatitis C virus. While few veterans of the Gulf Wars are yet in care for life-threatening illness, they too may have been exposed to chemical or biological agents. Combat experience is also associated with manifestations of PTSD. And, for yet unknown reasons, persons who served in the military, with any cohort, seem to be at significantly higher risk of ALS (amyotrophic lateral sclerosis), popularly called Lou Gehrig's disease. In fact, in 2008, amended VA regulations granted presumption of service connection to any veteran with the disease. This means that veterans with the disease are covered through the VA since the disease is considered connected to their prior military service.

Military service was for many individuals a major life-transforming experience. Many men and women have been changed by their combat and military experience, for better or for worse. Only by understanding that experience can mental health and health professionals provide the individualized and sensitive care veterans, as well as all other patients, so merit.

Editor's Note: Material from this section on veterans is drawn from PowerPoint presentations of Scott Shreve, Deborah Grassman, and Julie Phillips.

Kenneth J. Doka, PhD, MDiv, is a professor of gerontology at the Graduate School of The College of New Rochelle and senior consultant to the Hospice Foundation of America. Dr. Doka serves as editor of HFA's Living with Grief *book series, its* Journeys *newsletter, and numerous other books and publications. Dr. Doka has served as a panelist on HFA's* Living with Grief ® *video programs for 20 years. He is a past president of the Association for Death Education and Counseling (ADEC) and received an award for Outstanding Contributions in the field of Death Education. He is a member and past chair of the International Work Group on Death, Dying and Bereavement. In 2006, Dr. Doka was grandfathered in as a mental health counselor under New York's first state licensure of counselors. Dr. Doka is an ordained Lutheran minister.*

REFERENCES

Riley, M.W. (1987). On the significance of age in sociology. *American Sociological Review, 15,* 1-14.

Strauss, W., & Howe, N. (1991). *Generations: The history of America's future.* New York, NY: Quill.

Wright, A.A., & Katz, I.T. (2007). Letting go of the rope—aggressive treatment, hospice care, and open access. *New England Journal of Medicine, 357,* 324-327.

Special Issues in Treating Veterans at the End of Life

In Section I, we noted that military experience and participation in military culture has implications for end-of-life care. These implications are further explored in this section. We begin with Hallenbeck's chapter, as it provides an overview of the development of hospice and palliative care services within the Department of Veterans Affairs (VA). Hallenbeck notes the innovative role of the VA in the provision of hospice and palliative care; such services began in 1978, which was relatively early. In fact, the VA was one of the earliest systems to embrace the term palliative care. Hallenbeck also describes important lessons that the VA learned in the provision of such services. The first was that given the relatively large service area of VA facilities, home care, the predominant hospice model, was not really an option. This reality pushed the VA into another innovative role, providing hospice services within their nursing home facilities. Providing hospice and palliative services in this way emphasized the importance of the value of forging partnerships with community-based agencies.

Weller's chapter considers the impact of prior trauma on end-of-life care. Often at the end of life, clients engage in a life review, developing a coherent story of their life that reaffirms the meaningfulness of their existence. For those in combat, this life review can open old wounds, reminding them of traumatic events that caused spiritual or moral distress. Sometimes it may lead to the reemergence of the symptomatology of Posttraumatic Stress Disorder (PTSD). Weller offers both sound guidance on sensitively navigating life review and the need for end-of-life organizations treating veterans to be aware of the symptoms and resources for treating PTSD. Daniel's chapter reminds us that PTSD may also intersect with grief and that resources such as Vet Centers can assist clients in treating psychological issues.

Grassman's chapter follows. The violent nature of combat may not only create moral and spiritual distress but also engender a need for forgiveness.

This need is poignantly expressed not only in Grassman's chapter but in the *Voices* piece that so aptly illustrates that theme. Yet, we need to reiterate one theme implied in Grassman's chapter. Forgiveness is an issue only if it is an issue for a client. We never should impose our agenda on a patient. We do well to remember Shneidman's (1978) dictum that "no one needs to die in a state of psychoanalytic grace" (p. 211).

Periyakoil addresses another major issue mentioned earlier, that of pain management. In many ways, Periyakoil weaves together earlier themes. She notes the role that co-morbidity of conditions such as PTSD, psychological and spiritual distress, anxiety, or depression can play in complicating the management of pain. Periyakoil also describes how the culture of stoicism may create difficulties for assessing pain. It may be more effective to ask open-ended questions such as, "Are you comfortable?" rather than, "Are you in pain?" to moderate a stoical response. She is also aware that abuse of substances such as marijuana or prescription drugs may also inhibit effective pain management. Periyakoil's chapter provides sage guidance for navigating through these difficulties to manage pain. Yet, Quinlan's *Voices* piece reminds us of both the complexity of pain management in some cases with veterans, as well as another piece of Shneidman's (1978) wisdom; we often die as we lived.

The final pieces in this section reaffirm the resources that exist to assist veterans as they struggle with illness and death. Jones begins with a simple recognition that many veterans will receive care, including care at the end of life, in community-based facilities that may be unaware of the special needs or issues that veterans face, as well as the entitlements and benefits that may be available to support veterans. Jones offers a primer on the organization and benefits of the Veterans Administration, as well as a call for communication, collaboration, and coordination. Koepsell and staff members from the National Hospice and Palliative Care Organization (NHPCO) conclude with a description of a hospice-wide NHPCO-sponsored program, *We Honor Veterans*, which seeks to achieve that goal.

REFERENCE

Shneidman, E. (1978). Some aspects of psychotherapy with dying persons. In C. Garfield (Ed.), *Psychosocial care of the dying patient* (p. 201-218). New York, NY: McGraw-Hill.

CHAPTER 6

History of Hospice and Palliative Care in the Department of Veterans Affairs

James Hallenbeck

The history of hospice and palliative care in the Department of Veterans Affairs (VA) parallels that of the general population and is best understood in a broader historical context. Following founder Cicely Saunders' establishment of St. Christopher's Hospice in England in 1967, the first hospice/palliative care programs in North America were established in 1974 and 1975 in Montreal, New York, and Connecticut (Hallenbeck and McDaniel, 2009; Kastenbaum, 1997; Stoddard, 1978). Hospice programs then disseminated rapidly across the United States. The first hospice on the West Coast, Hospice of Marin, was established in Marin, California in 1975 (Stoddard, 1978). This was an important development for the eventual creation of the Medicare Hospice Benefit, which drew heavily on Hospice of Marin's experience in providing hospice care at home (Mor and Greer, 1988). Over the next few years various experiments in the provision of hospice care were undertaken within the VA, including two at two California VA facilities, the Wadsworth VA (now part of West Greater Los Angeles VA Health Care System) and VA Palo Alto Health Care System.

The Wadsworth program, entitled the Palliative Treatment Program (PTP), began operations in 1978. This pilot project initially consisted of five dedicated beds, a hospice consultation team, and a home care team. The inpatient program expanded to 12 beds in 1981 (Olsen and Wilson, 1982). Interest in these "early adopter" hospice programs began to attract attention from the federal government. The Health Care Financing Administration (HCFA) launched the National Hospice Study in 1979. The VA Central Office in Washington, DC similarly watched the development of efforts at Wadsworth with interest. Having authorized the creation of the Wadsworth program in

1978, VA Central Office also issued a directive limiting the creation of formal hospice units within the VA, until the Wadsworth project could be evaluated. Still, as Dr. Olsen (1982), the founder of the Wadsworth project, has written, "This directive, however, did not preclude the many existing activities directed toward the excellent care of terminally ill patients in other VA facilities." VA Central Office also funded research into outcomes related to the Wadsworth program, led by Robert Kane (1984), who published one of the earliest studies examining costs associated with hospice care.

The Wadsworth program was interesting in a number of regards. Its use of the term *palliative* in its title was way ahead of its time. The term *palliative care* had been coined only in 1974 by the founder of the Montreal Royal Victoria Palliative Care Service, Dr. Balfour Mount. Dr. Mount (1997) has written that the term came to him while shaving, as the word *hospice* had a negative connotation in French and Spanish, which was of great relevance in French-speaking Quebec. The VA did not begin broadly using the term palliative care until much later, in 2000, when this term was used in a national VA survey. The project was also very unusual in including a formal consultation team and a home care branch. Both were closely linked with the inpatient hospice program. Again, this was well ahead of its time within the VA and at large.

It is interesting to note that patient selection criteria included, "hav[ing] been diagnosed at the VA Wadsworth Hospital as being terminally ill and for whom *further active therapeutic intervention is no longer appropriate*" [italics from author] and "have a life expectancy of 6 months or less" (Olsen and Wilson, 1982). The choice of terminology regarding therapeutic interventions is unfortunate. Today, we would argue that hospice and palliative care provide very active interventions, albeit ones that may have shifted in line with the patient's changing medical status and expressed goals of care. It is somewhat surprising to see a statement regarding a six-month life-expectancy in the selection criteria. Hospice founder Cicely Saunders chafed at the notion that hospice care was exclusively for terminally ill patients with a short life expectancy (Hallenbeck and McDaniel, 2009). For example, in a letter to Dr. Walter Baechi in 1977, she wrote, "May I add that we believe very strongly that a Hospice is not only for dying and that this should never be part of its title" (Clark, 2005). In letters during the late 1970s and early 1980s she expressed regret at the narrow interpretation of hospice eligibility in the United States. It is not clear (at least to this author), where the notion that hospice care ought to be restricted to the last six months of life first arose; it certainly did not come from Saunders. Stoddard, in her book *The Hospice Movement* (1978), similarly makes no mention of a six-month standard for hospice admission. As most readers will know, this standard was later codified in standards for the Medicare Hospice Benefit in 1982. It is also interesting in retrospect to notice what was not incorporated into the formal Wadsworth patient selection criteria; acceptance of a palliative approach to care by the patient or proxy decision maker. Acceptance of a palliative approach to care was codified in the Medicare Hospice Benefit and later, mimicking this, in the VA criteria for hospice eligibility. It is not clear why such a criterion was not included in Wadsworth's criteria. Perhaps they presumed patient/proxy acceptance under the first, no "further active therapeutic intervention" standard. The Wadsworth palliative care project along with the Wadsworth VA facility was later consolidated into the VA Greater Los Angeles Health Care System.

One of those early VA "projects" mentioned by Dr. Olsen in his article also began in 1978 at the Menlo Park division of the Palo Alto Health Care System. Having studied the available literature, and having contacted evolving hospices in the San Francisco Bay Area, including Hospice of Marin, VA Palo Alto staff decided to open a three-bed hospice unit within their new nursing home, which was just then finishing construction and which opened in 1979. The Menlo Park campus, under the direction of Dr. Mark Graeber as Chief of Staff, was a haven for veterans from what were perceived as being disadvantaged groups, such as psychiatric patients, nursing home patients, and the homeless. When Dr. Graeber heard about hospice care for the dying, he felt the provision of such care would fit in perfectly to his greater mission. This small, unofficial project eventually grew into one of the largest hospice and palliative care programs in the VA system.

I go into this detail regarding this early history of one, then small, VA hospice program because I think it is in many ways illustrative of the more common history of hospice evolution in the VA system. More often than not hospice care emerged from VA nursing home care. Wadsworth was quite unusual in having a home care and consultative branch. For the most part, early nursing home-based hospice programs in the VA evolved out of the limelight. As was true for Palo Alto, admission criteria to the program were locally developed and informal. Officially, hospice beds and admissions were classified as nursing home beds. While some VA facilities developed dedicated bed sections or units, in many cases hospice care was provided on a "scatter bed" model; patients admitted to such beds were recognized as dying, but it was not always clear what special services such patients received or how such patients differed in care or characteristics from many non-hospice patients. More often than not, such early hospice programs, like most of their non-governmental counterparts, functioned and evolved quite independent of academic, hospital-based medicine. In the majority of cases, clinician training (of all disciplines) and research were not key components of these programs.

The evolution of hospice within the VA began to diverge from the greater American hospice movement following the creation of the Medicare Hospice Benefit. The Medicare Hospice Benefit, modeled in large part after Hospice of Marin, emphasized hospice care at home (Mor and Greer, 1988). The establishment of the benefit, which provided a much-needed funding mechanism for hospice care, resulted in a great blossoming of community hospice programs, focused in large part on care at home. Like most other healthcare systems at the time, the emphasis in the VA was on institutional care, although the VA also operated a limited number of outpatient clinics, most geographically close to acute care hospitals. The provision of home care by VA personnel was quite limited.

An ongoing challenge for the VA was, and is, how best to serve a diverse veteran population across the entire country. Many veterans live at a great distance from the nearest VA facility. The direct provision of home care by VA staff is a major logistical challenge. It thus makes some sense that the VA did not follow Medicare's lead to create VA community hospice programs. While a few VA facilities reportedly attempted this, for the most part the evolution of VA hospice and palliative care continued within VA institutions, particularly VA nursing homes, now called Community Living Centers (CLCs).

Because many of the VA nursing home-based hospice programs of the 1980s and 1990s operated informally out of VA nursing homes, it is difficult to state precisely how many existed or how many veterans were served within particular programs. VA databases during this time classified all hospice patients simply as nursing home residents. Some programs, like the one at Palo Alto, operated out of dedicated bed sections and evolved strong cultural and professional identities very much in sync with hospices in the community. Others had looser structures, often referred to as "scatter bed" models, in which hospice care was provided to residents, wherever they might reside in the nursing home, by consultants. Such informality had certain advantages, encouraging programmatic experimentation and discouraging bureaucratization. VA nursing home-based hospice programs differed significantly from their community counterparts in that they were relatively free from direct fiscal and hospice regulatory and accreditation pressures.

The VA provides care through an annual capitated system, not a per-diem system, as under Medicare. Each VA facility is paid a fixed amount of money for each veteran each year, based on a sophisticated data system called VERA (Veterans Equitable Resource Allocation System). Individual veterans are classified into one of several reimbursement categories with increased payments being made for veterans with greater or more complex needs. No discrete reimbursement category exists specific to hospice care. This is not unusual in the VA system. Reimbursement for each individual veteran's care is based on care provision over an entire year; it is not generally based on services received in a particular program. It is therefore difficult under the VA system for discrete programs to determine if they made a net positive fiscal contribution to the greater healthcare system.

Hospice programs operating under VA nursing home auspices were (and still are) surveyed under Joint Commission nursing home standards, not hospice standards. In large part this was because the Joint Commission in developing their hospice standards followed the lead of the Medicare Hospice Benefit in interpreting hospice as predominantly a home care service.

While the informality of VA hospice programs during this time had advantages, there were also downsides. Programmatic growth was highly dependent on local champions and local support. Significant variability existed in terms of the availability of hospice care and arguably the quality of care provided. In 1992 a series of VA directives were issued, mandating VA facilities to either directly provide or to ensure access to hospice care. As a 1996 Hospice Program Guide summarized these policies, "All veterans needing and choosing hospice care would be provided with that care either through the VA directly, or through coordinated referrals to community hospice resources" (Kizer, 1996). These directives were important in establishing formal expectations for hospice care. The Veterans Health Care Eligibility Act of 1996 mandated an assessment of the effectiveness and efficiency of VA hospice programs, which was then done. The findings of this study were published a few years later (Hickey et al., 1998).

The study found that in 1996, 145 of 148 responding VA medical centers reported active hospice programs. Sixty-five (45%) of these did not directly provide hospice care, but did refer to non-VA community hospices. Eighty

(55%) provided some hospice care within the facility. Most of these also referred to community hospices, although eight facilities (6%) reported only providing hospice care within the facility. The study estimated that 11,000 veterans received some form of hospice care that year, up 21% as compared to the prior year.

Fourteen facilities reported having dedicated hospice units for a total of 141 beds. More often, dedicated bed programs were part of larger units. Thirty-three VA facilities reported such programs for 206 beds. Most such units and programs were between five and ten beds.

In tandem with broader efforts, VA interest in hospice and palliative care expanded dramatically in the late 1990s. In 1998 a two-year Faculty Leaders Project was initiated with the support of the Robert Wood Johnson Foundation. Thirty physician faculty leaders were chosen from across VA facilities, provided protected time, and mentored by VA and non-VA physician leaders. Many of these faculty leaders are champions for hospice and palliative care in the VA today. The focus of this initiative was to support better resident training of physicians.

This initiative gave rise to the Training and Program Assessment for Palliative Care (TAPC) project in 2000 (Office of Geriatrics and Extended Care, 2001). This one-year project represented a novel collaboration between the VA Office of Geriatrics and Extended Care, programmatically in charge of clinical care nursing home, home care, and hospice services in the VA, and the Office of Academic Affiliations (OAA), which has responsibility for trainees for all healthcare disciplines. This project was broad in scope and had four objectives.

- The completion of a comprehensive survey of the availability of hospice and palliative care programs across the VA.
- The creation of an online toolkit to assist VA clinicians in the development of hospice and palliative care services.
- The creation of an interprofessional palliative care fellowship program.
- The creation of a palliative care online newsletter.

Like the earlier 1996 survey, findings were based on facility self-report. Key findings of the survey were:
- 97 (89%) of the 109 survey respondents reported that their facilities provide some manner of hospice and/or palliative care services.
- Most hospice and palliative care is provided in nursing home units.

- A vast majority (72%) of the programs serve less than 100 patients/year.
- 45 (41%) of 109 survey respondents reported that their facilities have a hospice or palliative care consult team.
- 37 (37%) of 99 respondents reported that their hospice/palliative care teams manage the patient's plan of care.
- 41 (38%) of 107 respondents reported that their hospice or palliative care programs conduct weekly team meetings.
- Cancer is the most frequently cited diagnosis.
- The majority (72%) of survey respondents indicated that their hospice or palliative care programs require a prognosis of 6 months or less.
- 29 (27%) of 108 survey respondents reported not having referred a veteran to a community/home hospice agency in the prior year.

The report identified certain deficiencies in hospice and palliative care programs. Few facilities required specialized training or demonstration of competencies. Training, when present, focused primarily on pain management and advance care planning. Few facilities provided training on care coordination between VA and community agencies, grief and bereavement, or communication skills. Perhaps most importantly, respondents generally felt that not all veterans who could benefit from palliative care consultation or hospice services actually received these services. Only 17% of respondents believed 80 or more percent of veterans needing services received them.

The TAPC survey demonstrated great variability in the availability of services across the VA and suggested equally great variability in associated training and clinical competence. The results provided an important impetus for broader efforts working to ensure greater equity of access and service delivery.

The creation of the Interprofessional Palliative Care Fellowship program represented a partnership between the Office of Academic Affiliations (OAA), which oversees VA training programs, and the Office of Geriatrics and Extended Care. In 2000 there was a growing recognition nationally that palliative care should be considered a formal medical subspecialty. While the drive toward formal subspecialty status revolved around physicians, in keeping with the tenets of hospice and palliative care, there was recognition that formal, advanced training for other core disciplines should also be available. And thus, this fellowship began. Six VA facilities were chosen to be fellowship sites. Funding for these original six sites is still ongoing a decade later. Training was approved for advanced fellows in medicine, nursing, social work, psychology, chaplaincy, and pharmacy. Not all training sites provided training in all disciplines, but all sites were required to provide training for non-physician clinicians. In many ways this program was ahead of its time in going beyond an appreciation for interprofessional/interdisciplinary clinical teamwork to a requirement for interprofessional training.

TAPC was quickly followed by VAHPC (VA Hospice and Palliative Care initiative) in 2001. This two-year project was a collaboration between the VA Office of Geriatrics and Extended Care (GEC), the National Hospice and Palliative Care Organization (NHPCO), and the Center for Advanced Illness Coordinated Care (CAICC). This initiative had two major objectives: 1) To strengthen ties and collaborative efforts between VA facilities and community hospices and 2) to expand the availability of hospice and palliative care services throughout the VA. The major outcome of the first objective was the promotion of Hospice-Veteran Partnerships between VA facilities and community organizations, especially hospice agencies. A toolkit on how to establish such partnerships was established and widely disseminated. Hospice-Veteran Partnerships were spearheaded by Diane Jones of the Ethos Consulting Group, who worked closely with VA GEC leadership on this and other ventures during this period. As a result of this effort, Hospice-Veteran Partnerships began springing up across the country.

Beyond local successes in the establishment of such partnerships, this effort gradually gave rise to important shifts in attitudes regarding hospice care for veterans. Through this and subsequent efforts, community hospice agencies became better able to appreciate the special needs of veterans at the end of life and the scope of that need. Many hospice advocates and leaders were shocked to learn that more veterans were dying annually than were all Americans dying of cancer. Community hospice knowledge gaps were identified regarding clinical care needs, for example, regarding the prevalence of Posttraumatic Stress Disorder (PTSD). For most community hospice agencies, the VA system was an opaque, confusing bureaucracy that was difficult to comprehend or navigate. Numerous conferences and educational events were held with community partners to address clinical and administrative issues such as VA eligibility, referral processes, and mechanisms for payment.

Clinicians in the VA also learned much through this process. Clinicians came to better understand that, despite their best efforts, optimal care for veterans often required collaboration with community agencies. In many cases, VA clinicians similarly had little understanding of the workings of community hospices with which they interacted. This initiative went a long way to move the relationship between community hospices and VA facilities from strained interaction to active collaboration toward a common mission.

The VAHPC initiative recognized a need for expansion of hospice and palliative care services within the VA. The TAPC survey had highlighted a need for formal VA guidance on hospice eligibility and clarification of expectations relative to the provision of palliative care consultation within the VA. The older requirements to provide or purchase some type of hospice care or consultation had clearly become outmoded. In 2002 a Veterans Health Administration Directive was issued on hospice and palliative care workload capture. This memorandum established for the first time formal criteria for hospice eligibility within the VA and defined palliative care. VA hospice eligibility intentionally mimicked Medicare Hospice eligibility criteria:

1. Diagnosed with a life-limiting illness;
2. Treatment goals focus on comfort rather than cure;
3. Life expectancy determined by a VA physician to be 6 months or less if the disease runs its normal course, consistent with the prognosis component of the Medicare hospice criteria; and
4. Accepts hospice care.

The memorandum also established a new code for tracking VA hospice workload within VA nursing homes, Treating Specialty Code 96. The creation of this code allowed centralized tracking of hospice workload.

In 2002 a major presentation was given to the National Leadership Board of the Veterans Health Administration, which made the case for an expansion of hospice and palliative care services. The presentation included findings from the TAPC survey, information on variability in the provision of hospice care across VA, and for the first time, data on the high cost of end-of-life care in VA. This presentation and related work did much to engender VHA leadership support for subsequent expansion efforts.

In 2003 another important directive was issued addressing palliative care consultation. This directive mandated that all VA facilities have a palliative care consultation team. In issuing such a requirement the VA was well ahead of many large healthcare organizations at that time. In order to ensure an interdisciplinary approach to care, the directive required physician, nurse, social work, and chaplain participation, as well as some administrative support. Palliative care consultation workload was required to be reported in a standardized fashion. Together with the 2002 workload directive, this directive established clear expectations for the performance of hospice and palliative care workload and created a mechanism that would enable standardized workload tracking.

The work over the first few years of the new millennium established a strong foundation for the expansion of hospice and palliative care services. This effort came to full fruition in the Comprehensive End-of-Life Care (CELC) initiative in 2009.

James Hallenbeck, MD, is an associate professor of medicine at Stanford University in the Division of General Medical Disciplines. He is Associate Chief of Staff for Extended Care and director of Palliative Care Services at VA Palo Alto Health Care System. He is board certified in Internal Medicine and Hospice and Palliative Medicine. He was the project chair for a national Veterans Affairs taskforce (TAPC) which worked to expand and improve palliative care throughout the VA. He is the hub-site director for a fellowship program in palliative care offered by the VA at six training sites across the country, called the Interprofessional Palliative Care Fellowship Program. Dr. Hallenbeck's academic interests in the area of palliative care have included physician education, non-pain symptom management, and cultural aspects of end-of-life care. He is the author of the book Palliative Care Perspectives *(Oxford University Press, 2003).*

REFERENCES

Clark, D. (2005). *Cicely Saunders founder of the Hospice Movement selected letters 1959-1999*. New York, NY: Oxford University Press.

Hallenbeck, J., & McDaniel, S. (2009). Palliative care and pain management in the United States. In R. Moore (Ed.), *Biobehavioral approaches to pain*, (pp. 493-513). New York, NY: Springer.

Hickey, E.C., Berlowitz, D.R., Anderson, J., Hankin, C., Hendricks, A., & Lehner, L. (1998, February). *The Veterans Hospice Care Study: An evaluation of VA hospice programs. Final Report.* Report Number MRR 97-004. Bedford, MA: Management Decision and Research Center, Health Services Research and Development Service, Edith Nourse Rogers Memorial Veterans Hospital.

Kane, R.L., Wales, J., Bernstein, L., Liebowitz, A., & Kaplan, S. (1984). A randomised controlled trial of hospice care. *Lancet*, *1*(8382), 890-894.

Kastenbaum, R. (1997). Hospice care in the United States. In C. Saunders & R. Kastenbaum (Eds.), *Hospice care on the international scene*, (pp. 101-113). New York, NY: Springer.

Kizer, K. (1996). Foreword, *VHA program guide 1140.10*. Washington, DC: VHA.

Mor, V., & Greer, D. (1988). *The hospice experiment.* Baltimore, MD: Johns Hopkins University Press.

Mount, B. (1997). The Royal Victoria Hospital Palliative Care Service: A Canadian experience. In C. Saunders & R. Kastenbaum, (Eds.), *Hospice care on the international scene,* (pp. 73-85). New York, NY: Springer.

National Defense Research Institute and RAND Health. (2005). *Analyzing—and influencing—how the Department of Veterans Affairs allocates its health care dollars.* Washington, DC: The RAND Corporation.

Office of Geriatrics and Extended Care, Office of Academic Affiliations. (2001). *Toolkit for developing hospice and palliative care programs in the Department of Veterans Affairs Medical Centers.* Washington, DC: Veterans Health Administration.

Olsen, E., & Wilson, D. (1982). Hospice: Within the VA Hospital System. *Family & Community Health,* 5(3), 21-29.

Stoddard, S. (1978). *The Hospice Movement.* Briar Cliff Manor, NY: Stein and Day.

VA Palo Alto Hospice. (1978). Planning meeting notes. Palo Alto, CA: Author.

Veterans Health Administration Directive 10-92-001 (1992). Plans for Hospice Care of the Terminally Ill Veteran.

Veterans Health Administration Directive 10-92-050. (1992). Policy on Implementation of Hospice Consultation.

Veterans Health Administration Directive 10-92-092. (1992). Policy on Implementation of Hospice Programs.

Coping with Trauma and Posttraumatic Stress Disorder (PTSD) at Life's End: Managing Life Review

Ryan Weller

Meet Frank, a military veteran who is at home receiving hospice care. His time left to live is likely days to weeks, and he is now so weak that he spends all of his time in a hospital bed in the living room. He is not just passively lying there; he spends most of his time thinking back over his life. Some of his memories are pleasant, like fun times in his childhood with his friends. Other memories bring pain and regret, like his first marriage that did not go so well. But where do his three years in the Air Force fit into his life story? For some, time spent in the military can be a proud experience, full of memories that have been shared freely for years. For others, it is the hardest period in life to stop thinking about. In Frank's case, it is the hardest period in his life to know where to *begin* thinking.

Assisting veterans who want to engage in *life review*, which means talking about their memories and the meaning they give to the events in their life, is a privilege. Knowing how to support a veteran who is undergoing life review can be uniquely challenging. The purpose of this chapter is to assist the family member, friend, caregiver, or clinician in their life review conversations with veterans who have experienced trauma in military service. To better understand military-related trauma, the first section of this chapter gives an overview of different types of distress, including Posttraumatic Stress Disorder (PTSD). The second section offers guidance on navigating these conversations with veterans who choose to share and reflect on their lives which, for many, will be for the first time.

TRAUMA AND POSTTRAUMATIC STRESS DISORDER (PTSD)

Exposure to trauma and living with the subsequent post-exposure aftermath has likely always been associated with military service, although it has not always been labeled and defined as it is today. In the American Civil War era, traumatized veterans were said to have "irritable heart." Many World War I veterans were labeled as having "shell shock." In World War II, nervous veterans were said to be afflicted with "battle fatigue" or "neurosis." Since 1980, the psychiatric community has formally recognized these conditions as Posttraumatic Stress Disorder (American Psychiatric Association, 1980). Many veterans have experienced trauma or lived through harrowing conditions but have not had their lives adversely affected. Other trauma survivors have struggled to live a life that is integrated with society at all and may have a formal PTSD diagnosis. There is a third category of veterans who may not have been diagnosed with PTSD, but are still bothered by experiences with trauma or distress. This section of the chapter will review the emotional, spiritual, and psychological damage from different types of trauma: moral distress, spiritual distress, memories of living in a hostile environment, or exposure to violence, in addition to living with a formal diagnosis of PTSD.

Moral distress

The military experience can place soldiers in situations where they must perform or bear witness to behavior that is in conflict with their personal morals. Litz et al. (2009) use this definition for "morally injurious experiences: perpetrating, failing to prevent, bearing witness to, or learning about acts that transgress deeply held moral beliefs and expectations" (p. 700). The memories of these experiences can be uncomfortable to the point of distraction or distress, and they can be the source of regret or despair throughout life. This can be experienced acutely as veterans approaching life's end reflect on their military experience. Moral distress can be associated with feelings of guilt or shame. There can also be a strong component of fear of judgment by others. As with other forms of trauma, these feelings and fears can block veterans from sharing their stories with others. Some veterans with PTSD will have a strong component of moral distress as a part of their traumatic experience(s), however, many more veterans live with moral distress who do not meet criteria for PTSD.

Case example

Mr. G is a World War II army veteran. He served honorably for three years and was primarily stationed in Europe and North Africa. As he approached the end of his life, Mr. G was an enthusiastic storyteller about his time in military service. However, there was one subject that he said was still bothering him and keeping him up at night. He believed there was no justification for American involvement in the European war theatre, and therefore he felt that the acts of violence he had to commit there were unjust. "I had no problem with the Germans. I was mad at the Japanese. They were the ones who bombed us. The Germans didn't do anything to us. I couldn't believe I was being sent over to Europe. I enlisted to go fight the Japanese, and I got sent to fight the Germans. I just didn't feel right about that, and I still don't."

Spiritual distress

Similar to moral distress, spiritual distress is living with memories of behavior that are incongruent with one's religious or spiritual beliefs. Feelings of regret, shame, guilt, and fear are also associated with spiritual distress. Some veterans leave military service with spiritual beliefs intact or strengthened, and they may find peace, resolution, and forgiveness through prayer or discussion with a leader in their faith tradition. Others leave military service with much disruption to their spiritual beliefs. They may strongly question the existence of God after witnessing atrocities on Earth and wonder, "Where was God in this? Why wasn't this stopped? I prayed for this to end, but was my prayer not heard?"

When previously held religious beliefs are no longer held or are questioned, it can be difficult for some and impossible for others to find meaning and reconciliation within those same beliefs. However, that does not mean the search for understanding and meaning ends. Fontana and Rosenheck (2004), writing about veterans' spiritual distress and PTSD, state, "...veterans' motivation for continued pursuit of mental health services does not appear to be primarily greater symptom relief or more social contact. Rather...a primary motivation of veterans' continuing pursuit of treatment is their search for a meaning and purpose to their traumatic experiences" (p. 582).

As veterans approach the end of life, the urgency to find meaning can be intensified. Some will be distressed by a fear of judgment by God for behavior committed during military service. Others will question the existence of God completely and will anxiously wonder what the afterlife will be like or doubt that there will be an afterlife at all. Many will not speak about these concerns at all, but may appear aloof, removed, anxious, cranky, or tearful; clinicians need to consider that these veterans may in fact be experiencing spiritual distress.

Case example

Mr. B is a 66-year-old Vietnam veteran who was drafted into service in 1968. He had just begun dating a girl in his town and regularly attended her family's Quaker church. Just as he was beginning to develop his beliefs about pacifism, he was drafted. Members of the church tried to help him receive conscientious objector status, but since he had a short history in the church, it was denied by his local draft board. While in service, Mr. B experienced intense emotional reactions to participating in the killing of enemy soldiers and even, inadvertently, many civilians. Following his time in service, Mr. B married his high school girlfriend and continued a lifetime of involvement in the Quaker church. However, he never felt comfortable discussing the violence he committed or witnessed in Vietnam. As he entered what was his last weeks of life, he felt like he was "bursting" with guilt over taking others' lives and "not trying harder to get discharged or sent somewhere else." He died believing God forgave him, but he never gave indication that he forgave himself.

Trauma from a hostile environment

Prolonged exposure to a hostile environment, even without experiencing or witnessing violence, is in itself a traumatic experience. Fontana and Rosenheck (1999) describe elements of a "malevolent environment" (p. 118) that veterans may have experienced, including horrendous weather, exposure to dangerous insects and animals, insufficient supplies, starvation, and lack of shelter. Living under the threat of violence or learning of the death of a comrade also contributes to a hostile environment. King, King, Gudanowski, and Vreven (1995) state that of all stressors that contribute to PTSD, a "malevolent environment appeared to be the most potent factor for men and women" (p. 192) who served in Vietnam. In the later stages of life, there can be both psychological and physical reminders of exposure to a hostile environment. For example, suffering from frostbite injuries received during service in cold conditions in Eastern Europe can manifest and bring back both physical pain and also agonizing memories of living in freezing conditions.

Case example

Mr. J is a veteran of the Korean War. He lived in a prisoner-of-war camp for several months and experienced exposure to both extremely hot and cold weather. The food he was served came at unpredictable times and was not familiar to him; he was surrounded by rats, cockroaches, and other insects. He had to live without knowing much about the status of the war, his buddies, or his family back home. Fifty years later, as his death came within weeks, Mr. J began hoarding his medication. He would tuck the pain medication that his wife gave him inside his cheek and then later grip the pills in his hand until he could hide them inside his bedside drawer. This continued until he was too weak to access his drawer. His hospice nurse, who came to his house to assess his spouse's report of increased grimacing and pain, found a tight fist holding two days' worth of pain medicine. Mrs. J stated she never noticed her husband hoard anything before, but now as he became increasingly debilitated and dependent on others for his care, some of the survival tactics that he learned as a POW returned.

Trauma from exposure to violence

Military experience can include witnessing, committing, or receiving violent acts. Violence can be in the form of physical violence or killing, but also as other atrocities such as sexual assault or mutilation. Breslau and Davis (1987) found that between 73% and 93% of Vietnam veterans experienced " 'enemy fire,' 'buddy killed in action,' 'combat patrol and other dangerous missions,' 'surrounded by the enemy,' and 'witnessed atrocities' " (p. 581). It is important to note that violent acts occur not only during wartime combat between enemy soldiers, but also during peacetime hostilities and between soldiers of the same service unit. Exposure to violence can be powerful enough to have a negative, transgenerational impact on veterans' families. An increase in behavioral disturbances in children of Vietnam War veterans, 15 to 20 years after the veterans' exposure to violence, was noted by Rosenheck and Fontana (1998).

Case example

Mr. P is a veteran of the Vietnam War. While serving in Vietnam, Mr. P was a gunner who had the duty of clearing enemy villages of Viet Cong presence. He left service not knowing how many enemy combatants he had killed nor how many civilian adults and children were in the crossfire. He married, had one son, and divorced. He had frequent nightmares and flashbacks to his time clearing these villages. Being present with his son was at times extremely difficult and painful for him as he would be lost in these memories. He was not always kind to his son as a result, and drinking alcohol seemed to be the easiest form of medication to ease his anxiety. His son was arrested twice for shoplifting and was suspended from school frequently for fighting on the playground. Mr. P and his son lost touch over the years. As Mr. P approached death, the hospice social worker tried to honor his request to find his son, but to his surprise discovered the son, while trying to hold up a convenience store, had been killed. After informing Mr. P that his son was dead, the veteran held back some tears and never spoke of him again.

Posttraumatic Stress Disorder (PTSD)

The fourth edition of the Diagnostic and Statistical Manual of Mental Disorders (DSM-IV) (American Psychiatric Association, 1994), categorizes PTSD as anxiety disorder characterized by a traumatic event where actual or threatened death or physical harm was experienced or witnessed. The DSM-IV lists numerous possible symptoms, such as: recurrent and intrusive thoughts or dreams; avoiding thoughts, feelings, or activities and places that may trigger memories of the trauma; signs of increased arousal (difficulty with sleep, irritable mood, hypervigilance, and strong startle reflex). The symptoms must be present for more than one month to meet criteria for diagnosis, and it needs to cause significant distress or impairment in social functioning.

As most would expect, instances of PTSD are higher in the veteran population than in the civilian population. In the general public, 3.6% of men and 9.7% of women have a lifetime prevalence of PTSD. Vietnam veterans have a 30.9% lifetime prevalence among men and 26% among women. It is estimated that 13.8% of veterans from the Iraq and Afghanistan wars meet criteria for PTSD (Gradus, accessed 2012). However, many more veterans have experienced trauma or feel distress from trauma exposure but do not meet the formal diagnostic criteria for PTSD. PTSD can also be misdiagnosed as another anxiety disorder or as depression.

PTSD can be acute or chronic, and veterans are more likely to experience delayed-onset PTSD than civilians (Andrews, Brewin, Philpott, and Stewart, 2007). It is not uncommon for family members to be unaware that their loved one has PTSD, and to discover it for the first time as the veteran transitions closer to debilitation or death. Symptoms of PTSD may increase as disability increases and coping skills decline (Hamilton and Workman, 1998). When PTSD symptoms have acute manifestation at the end of life, this can be alarming, confusing, and distressing to families. It is important for hospice staff to be prepared to provide education to families about PTSD.

As stated by Feldman and Periyakoil (2006), treatment options for PTSD in a hospice or palliative care setting can be limited by several factors. First, hospice staff may not have trauma experts available to manage the symptoms. Second, if a patient with a prognosis of weeks is experiencing acute-onset

PTSD, there may not be time for pharmacologic intervention to take effect. Third, veterans with PTSD may not have the necessary trust in their medical providers to accept interventions. Likewise, distrust and avoidance behavior can explain why some veterans approach death without any family or friends in their lives. Without trust from the patient or the presence of any family or friends to encourage that trust, the providers must use what Feldman and Periyakoil (2006, p. 217) call "an extremely patient-centered approach," where the relationship between provider and patient is "egalitarian" and patient control is enhanced.

Case example

Mr. F is a 77-year-old veteran of the Korean War. He never married and lived most of the last 20 years of his life in a small trailer park outside of the city. He refused to see a physician until the owner of the trailer park persuaded him to come to the local VA emergency department to evaluate a very large tumor that was growing on the side of his face. When he checked into the emergency room, Mr. F entered "None" as his next of kin. Mr. F was briefly hospitalized, but was released to a nursing facility once he made it clear he would not accept any treatment for this rapidly growing, malignant tumor. It was not easy to get Mr. F to agree to be admitted to the nursing home, and he only did so after the trailer park owner told him he could not come back to live alone in a trailer.

Mr. F was fairly irritable with staff at the nursing home, but overall adjusted to his new surroundings. However, staff noted many unusual behaviors. At specific hours of the day Mr. F would get out of bed, look under his bed, look in his closet, look out the window, and down the hallway. Staff had to announce themselves loudly from the doorway before entering, because one time he took a swing at a nurse who was near his bed when he woke up. Staff and other residents became very concerned when Mr. F began screaming at different intervals during the day and even occasionally at night. Eventually a nurse realized he was screaming whenever a plane flew overhead. Although by this point Mr. F was too delirious to confirm this, staff assumed the sound of the planes triggered flashbacks. A simple intervention of providing him earplugs helped block that trigger, although staff had to continue to be cautious when approaching him for any physical care. Even in his last hours of life he was strong and would occasionally swing or swat at those trying to bathe him.

LIFE REVIEW WHEN TRAUMA IS A PART OF THE STORY

Life review is the process of self-reflection and evaluation of a life that, in the context of a hospice setting, is approaching the end. Life review can be conducted internally and in silence, or can be shared with families, clinical staff, or caregivers. It can be a transformative experience for some, helping them to reach a point of "forgiveness for self and others" (Jenko, Gonzalez, and Seymour, 2007, p. 165). Butler (1963) described life review as "a naturally occurring, universal mental process characterized by the progressive return to consciousness of past experiences, and, particularly, the resurgence of unresolved conflicts; simultaneously, and normally, these revived experiences and conflicts can be surveyed and reintegrated" (p. 66). When trauma (and associated feelings of guilt, shame, and regret) is a part of the life story, however, the life review process can be excruciatingly painful. It can also be difficult if not impossible to reintegrate the trauma experience(s).

Approaching veterans about life review

Just as no one person is the same as another, no veteran is the same as another veteran. However, it can be helpful to consider some similar experiences that many veterans share. For some, their time in the military was memorable but has not really impacted their post-service life. For others, time in the military was a key highlight in their lives and perhaps the most significant contribution made in their lifetime. Veterans have all had some degree of military training that likely included training related to controlling one's emotions and emphasizing a stoic response to pain or suffering (Hoyt, Rielage, and Williams, 2011). This training can manifest at the end of life, which can result in physical pain being denied and emotional pain being stifled. It is important to remember that suffering may be happening even if there are no outward signs of it.

Veterans may not want to talk about their military experience, perhaps because of the trauma associated with it or perhaps because it is not the most significant piece of their life story. However, others have come to believe or experience that family and friends do not have the interest, or perhaps the fortitude, to hear their story. Other veterans do not want to share their story and risk being judged or rejected for its contents. Simply asking, "I understand you served in the military. What was that experience like for you?" is likely to bring about some sort of response. The response may be indifferent, glowing, or hostile but, more likely than not, the response will be genuine. By bringing up the topic, the process has begun to engage the veteran in his or her story.

The duration of the life review process may be one brief visit or perhaps a few, but time is unpredictable given the short prognosis and possibility of slipping into delirium or unconsciousness prior to death. It is important for caregivers and staff to engage hospice patients in life review when the opportunity is right, because there may not be a second chance.

Theoretical guidance

In the mental health field, no one theory or model of psychotherapy has been proven to be most effective in the treatment of PTSD (Benish, Imel, and Wampold, 2007; Wampold et al., 2010). However, the opportunity to share about their traumatic experiences has been reported to be helpful by most who experienced trauma (Zatzick et al., 2001). Recently, much attention is being given to the usefulness of Narrative Therapy and Narrative Exposure Therapy in the treatment of PTSD and also to the process of conducting life review (Bohlmeijer, Westerhof, and Emmerick-de Jong, 2008; Korte, Bohlmeijer, Cappeliez, Smit, and Westerhof, 2012; Robjant and Fazel, 2010). Narrative Therapy, as developed by White and Epston (1990), is a type of counseling which helps patients or clients reconstruct and expand their view of their personal history and identity. The theory assumes that people view their lives like a story, and they retain or reject experiences depending on how well they fit with their dominant storyline. As partners, the client and counselor discuss in detail the patient's existing story and then rebuild the story while integrating new alternatives, views, and experiences which have been left out previously.

When working with veterans who are in the last weeks or months of life, it is often not possible to engage them in formal Narrative Therapy or other psychotherapeutic processes that would be done in a counseling office or with a specific curriculum conducted over a set number of weeks. Instead, it can be helpful to borrow certain components of narrative therapy that can be utilized as tools to assist with life review.

1. Realize that life review is not about collecting facts or eyewitness accounts, but understanding the life story from the perspective of the patient (Kropf and Tandy, 1998).
2. To better understand the story, ask questions that are open-ended and may have a hint of wonderment. "I heard you say that many soldiers on the enemy side died because of your work as a gunner. I know this has been on your mind ever since. I was wondering, what thoughts do you have about the people whose lives were actually saved because of that same work?"

3. Be prepared to reflect back to the patient items that sounds like contradictions in their story. "I am a little confused. You said that nothing good came from your time in the service. But you just mentioned how you were able to get closer to your son by teaching him some of the survival techniques you learned from the service. Is that something good that came from your military experience?"

4. Anticipate that some patients will surprise themselves with some memories that they have forgotten or failed to integrate in their life story until now. "You know, I forgot all about that praying I did when I was over there. I remember asking God that if it's His will for me to stay and fight, then so be it. Back then it seemed like God didn't hear my prayers. Now I wonder if that was just what He wanted me to be doing."

5. It is not enough to listen to the life story and ask questions that bring to light forgotten or nonintegrated memories; the counselor should also reflect back to the patient their new story. With healthier patients, this is often done in the form of a letter that summarizes their story with the newly discovered elements incorporated. For a patient at the end of life, a verbal recount is likely the only option.

DEALING WITH INTENSE EMOTIONS AND STORIES

It is not easy to bear witness to the stories of others, particularly when the stories involve violence or tragedy. It can be anguishing to see another suffer and know that this person has been suffering from these experiences for many years. Being present in silence can often be the best way to demonstrate to the veteran that his or her story, no matter how horrific, did not cause the listener to reject him or become so overwhelmed that she could no longer share. The listener should not try to rush the veteran along or quiet the story with well-intended phrases like, "Well, it's okay now, that happened a long time ago," when to the veteran it feels like it is happening now and not 50 years ago. It is okay to be silent and to listen; when the story is over, it may be the right time to offer words of reassurance or even forgiveness. "Thank you for sharing that with me. I know that wasn't easy to talk about. I want you to know that I respect you all the more knowing now what you have carried with you since the war. I'd like to hear more if there is more you want to share."

Just as the physical effort of caring for someone who is terminally ill can be significant, so too can be the emotional effort. It is important for those who are privileged to listen to a life review that involves trauma to make the effort to care for themselves. If you have just absorbed a story of high intensity, what do you do with that? Think about it while walking in the sunshine. Release it through prayer or meditation. Share about it with your fellow team members. It is important to have a plan for self-care to strengthen and sustain oneself, because the need to bear witness to more intense stories may come again soon.

WHAT TO HOPE FOR FROM LIFE REVIEW?

Some people say that people die the way they lived. This adage denies the transformative process that can happen at the end of life for many. Providing a veteran with the opportunity to reflect on his or her life can be the key to a transformative experience when life expectancy is very short. Life review can be intense and frightening for the veteran and, sometimes, for the one privileged to bear witness to the veteran's story. What can be gained from doing this when life expectancy is short? For the veteran, the sharing of the story in itself can be cathartic. From sharing, reflecting, and learning new insights, some may come to a place of forgiveness (of themselves or others) or internal rest that they did not experience before. For the family, this can be an opportunity to learn more about their loved one, and can give the family new insights into not only the veteran but also how his or her life experiences affected the entire family. For the bedside clinician, what can be gained is the feeling of privilege and honor that comes from being trusted with these stories and facilitating an experience of support and acceptance before the veteran dies.

Editor's Note: The views expressed in this chapter do not necessarily express the views of the Department of Veterans Affairs or the United States Government.

Ryan Weller, *LCSW, is the Palliative Care Program Manager for the Department of Veterans Affairs Northwest Network (VISN 20). Since 2002 he has been the coordinator of the Palliative Care Consult Team at the Portland VA Medical Center (PVAMC) and is on the faculty of the PVAMC's Interprofessional Fellowship in Palliative Care. Mr. Weller is a member of the Oregon Hospice Association board of directors and serves as a columnist for the Journal of Palliative Medicine social media portal. His commitment to hospice and palliative care began in 1995 when he started a year of working and training with Wellspring Hospice-At-Home in London, England.*

REFERENCES

American Psychiatric Association. (1980). *Diagnostic and statistical manual of mental disorders* (3rd ed.). Washington, DC: American Psychiatric Association.

American Psychiatric Association. (1994). *Diagnostic and statistical manual of mental disorders* (4th ed.). Washington, DC: American Psychiatric Association.

Andrews, B., Brewin, C.R., Philpott, R., & Stewart, L. (2007). Delayed-onset posttraumatic stress disorder: A systematic review of the evidence. *American Journal of Psychiatry, 164*(9), 1319-1326.

Benish, S.G., Imel, Z.E., & Wampold, B.E. (2007). The relative efficacy of bona fide psychotherapies for treating post-traumatic stress disorder: A meta-analysis of direct comparisons. *Clinical Psychology Review (28)*, 746-758.

Bohlmeijer, E.T., Westerhof, G.J., & Emmerick-de Jong, M. (2008). The effects of integrative reminiscence on meaning in life: Results of a quasi-experimental study. *Aging and Mental Health, 12*(5), 639-646.

Breslau, N., & Davis, G.C. (1987). Posttraumatic stress disorder: The etiologic specificity of wartime stressors. *American Journal of Psychiatry, 144*(5), 578-583.

Butler, R. (1963). The life review: An interpretation of reminiscence. *Psychiatry, 26*, 65-76.

Feldman, D., & Periyakoil, V.S. (2006). Posttraumatic stress disorder at the end of life. *Journal of Palliative Medicine, 9*(1), 213-218.

Fontana, A., & Rosenheck, R. (1999). A model of war zone stressors and posttraumatic stress disorder. *Journal of Traumatic Stress, 12*(1), 111-125.

Fontana, A., & Rosenheck, R. (2004). Trauma, change in strength of religious faith, and mental health service use among veterans treated for PTSD. *Journal of Nervous and Mental Disease, 192*(9), 579-584.

Gradus, J. (accessed September 24, 2012). Epidemiology of PTSD. http://www.ptsd.va.gov/

Hamilton, J.D., & Workman, R.H. (1998). Persistence of combat-related posttraumatic stress symptoms for 75 years. *Journal of Traumatic Stress, 11*(4), 763-768.

Hoyt, T., Rielage, J.K., & Williams, L.F. (2011). Military sexual trauma in men: A review of reported rates. *Journal of Trauma and Dissociation, 12,* 244-260.

Kropf, N.P., & Tandy, C. (1998). Narrative therapy with older clients: The use of a meaning-making approach. *Clinical Gerontologist, 18*(4), 3-16.

Litz, B.T., Stein, N., Delaney, E., Lebowitz, L., Nash, W.P., Silva, C., & Maguen, S. (2009). Moral injury and moral repair in war veterans: A preliminary model and intervention strategy. *Clinical Psychology Review, 29,* 695-706.

Jenko, M., Gonzalez, L., & Seymour, M.J. (2007). Life review with the terminally ill. *Journal of Hospice and Palliative Nursing, 9*(3), 159-167.

King, D.W., King, L.A., Gudanowski, D.M., & Vreven, D.L. (1995). Alternative representations of war zone stressors: Relationships to posttraumatic stress disorder in male and female Vietnam veterans. *Journal of Abnormal Psychology, 104*(1), 184-196

Korte, J., Bohlmeijer, E.T., Cappeliez, P., Smit, F., & Westerhof, G.J. (2012). Life review therapy for older adults with moderate depressive symptomatology: A pragmatic randomized controlled trial. *Psychological Medicine, 42*(6), 1163-1173.

Robjant, K., & Fazel, M. (2010). The emerging evidence for narrative exposure therapy: A review. *Clinical Psychology Review, 30,* 1030-1039.

Rosenheck, R., & Fontana, A. (1998). Transgenerational effects of abusive violence on the children of Vietnam combat veterans. *Journal of Traumatic Stress, 11*(4), 731-741.

Wampold, B.E., Imel, Z.E., Laska, K.M., Benish, S., Miller, S., Fluckiger, C.,... Budge, S. (2010). Determining what works in the treatment of PTSD. *Clinical Psychology Review, 30,* 923-933.

White, M., & Epston, D. (1990). *Narrative means to therapeutic ends.* New York, NY: W.W. Norton & Co.

Zatzick, D.F., Kang, S.M., Hinton, W.L., Kelly, R.H., Hilty, D.M., Franz, C.E.,...Kravitz, R.L. (2001). Posttraumatic concerns: A patient-centered approach to outcome assessment after traumatic physical injury. *Medical Care, 39*(4), 327-339.

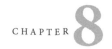

Grief and Traumatic Stress: Conceptualizations and Counseling Services for Veterans

Lori R. Daniels

For someone diagnosed with Posttraumatic Stress Disorder (PTSD), the complexities of emotionally juggling traumatic stress symptoms while simultaneously facing strong emotions associated with grief and loss can be overwhelming and trigger trauma-related reactions. Neria and Litz (2004) summarize this dilemma while describing the interplay of grief response and traumatic stressors: "Typically, loss by traumatic means (e.g., homicide) is conceptualized as a traumatic stressor event than can lead to posttraumatic stress disorder (PTSD)... However, grief is a distinct individual, social, and relational experience" (p. 73).

What hospice or palliative care providers may observe with some of their war veterans or traumatized patients are some of the more commonly reported PTSD symptoms: problematic sleep, acting out of past memories, nightmares related to traumatic event(s), increased feelings of being unsafe, irritability, low self-esteem, and anxiety related to diminished control of their environment. Add to these struggles impending or anticipated loss and these symptoms may worsen significantly. Some hospice workers describe hearing a spontaneous disclosure of a veteran's traumatic event near the end of life when previous information about other significant war incidents had not been shared (personal communication, June 24, 2011). The appearance of a veteran's problems can seem convoluted or nonsensical to the untrained provider, when, in fact, this type of response is more typical for trauma survivors who are faced with future losses. One way to look at this interplay between grief and traumatic stressors is to consider unresolved grief as a part of a survivor's traumatic stress response, and traumatic stress as a form of complicated grief. The following section is an effort to make sense of the resurgence of traumatic stress symptoms that can appear around impending loss and unresolved grief responses in veterans, and to discuss the role of VA medical centers and Vet Centers in providing grief counseling.

INTERRELATIONSHIP BETWEEN TRAUMATIC EVENTS AND GRIEF

Depending on the traumatic event situation, there are tangible and intangible losses that occur very quickly during a traumatic incident. Tangible losses may include the loss of life, limbs, personal possessions; intangible losses may include the loss of a relationship, a dream of the future, a role in life, or the ability to trust others. At the time of crisis, war trauma survivors, as well as non-war veterans who are victimized by violence, are often faced with a sudden and overwhelming flood of information, which they must quickly sift through in order to make split-second decisions for survival. Unfortunately, many of these decisions are focused on making choices between the "lesser of two evils," without a fully satisfactory outcome. Active-duty service members are often in situations where they cannot reflect on the choices made during a crisis. This reality may be due to competing demands of being in a war zone, or they may choose not to access resources if they have self-evaluated their decision as being not acceptable or even shameful (Neria and Litz, 2004).

Thus begins the complications and challenges of trauma survivors who are also dealing with more recent or current losses. Because traumatic stress and grief responses are inextricably connected, a possible helpful task for providers lies in determining the context of current loss(es) with past loss(es) for veteran trauma survivors.

Context of grieving prior to traumatic events from the military

What determines how a patient copes after a traumatic event appears to be related to his or her pre-trauma experiences with grief and loss. Service members who have never learned to grieve prior to experiencing a traumatic event in the military or were traumatized during their childhood may consider normal grieving as an abnormal response. Learning about pre-military losses and past coping skills from a veteran's history provides the context of how he or she may have emotionally treated a traumatic event loss during active duty, as well as current or impending losses. By understanding more about a patient's past and current losses (whether traumatic or not), hospice and healthcare professionals are able to approach veteran patients (or their family) with better perspective and expectations. In addition, considering the possible reactivation of traumatic stress symptoms when losses re-trigger PTSD, workers can consider alternative resources to assist a veteran with these issues, normalize the changes, and offer appropriate support.

It is possible that trauma survivors diagnosed with PTSD respond differently to recent losses than those who have not experienced a traumatic event (Green, 2000; Raphael, 1997). Survivors dealing with sudden or unpredictable tragedy may be less likely to access emotions that permit them to regain a sense of normality and health in order to move forward with their lives. When these individuals have a difficult time adjusting, they may be at higher risk for a response comparable to complicated grief (Monk, Houck, and Shear, 2006). This can occur if survivors are unable to communicate their emotions experienced as a result of a traumatic event, especially thoughts about their own role during the incident. Aspects of one's trauma experience may remain hidden.

In addition, one study found that survivor perceptions of enduring causal influences as factors within experiencing a traumatic event (instead of attributing a catastrophic experience as an isolated incidence) are significantly related to PTSD symptoms (Gray and Lombardo, 2004). In other words, part of whether previous trauma is considered a random or isolated event or a part of one's persisting experience of life (a bleak or fatalistic perspective) contributes to whether people have PTSD or not. Another study also found that those who explained their own personal traumatic events as occurrences that were attributed to their own internal beliefs about victimization were also more likely to have PTSD (Falsetti and Resick, 1995).

Should survivor thoughts be focused on feeling responsible for a tragic outcome, a survivor may opt to not share this information with others (e.g., "I should have stopped him from getting in the car" or "I should have been there when the accident occurred because I would have done something different and they'd still be alive"). Self-blaming thoughts such as these can result in an emotional dilemma of feeling excessively responsible for a negative outcome, lack of control to change the outcome, and an unwillingness to reveal self-blaming thoughts to others for fear of rejection. Self-blaming or victimizing beliefs are then never challenged, since a trauma survivor has not communicated this struggle with others, or minimizes the impact of the incident. By maintaining the secrecy of self-blame (e.g., "I'm powerless," "I'm not a good person after what I've done," or "If you knew what've I've seen or done, you wouldn't want to talk with me"), many survivors with PTSD will withdraw and isolate themselves from their social supports and have continued chronic problems.

A survivor's response to loss often depends on past experiences of loss. Although there is little empirical study conducted on the mediators of traumatic bereavement, some have suggested that previous experience of trauma or significant previous loss may prolong the grieving process, potentially leading to more problematic symptoms after the loss of a significant other (Neria and Litz, 2004; Green, 2000; Raphael, 1997). Those struggling with bereavement responses may make assumptions about what grief actually looks like, deny any experience of grieving, consider normal grieving as an abnormal response, feel inordinately uncomfortable around those who express grief-related sadness, or defer grief to others. If a survivor's experience of loss was in the context of serving in the U.S. military in a war zone, when the ability to grieve was not an option due to a crisis situation, the ability to access emotions appropriate for the loss will be far more challenging (Neria and Litz, 2004).

Taking into account the severity and intensity of traumatic occurrences, those who experience these events without knowing how to cope with loss are more challenged in regards to their readjustment after a traumatic event. This is illustrated in the case of Mr. Z, who was active-duty during the Vietnam War for one year. He was in the Navy, but found himself attached to a Marine Corps unit for his job, something he was not anticipating. As a result of his reassignment, he was treated differently by the Marines, and felt ostracized for "not being one of them" due to his ethnic background, as well as being from another branch of the military. One particular traumatic incident involved the death of a civilian, and Mr. Z felt a heightened sense of responsibility for this particular outcome. For years, he refused to discuss the incident for fear that anyone who knew what happened would reject him. In addition, he also was demonstrating classic PTSD symptoms, including recurrent nightmares. Through psychotherapy, Mr. Z finally revealed his self-blaming thoughts about the civilian's death, using phrases and descriptions that also indicated some losses that occurred within him. "I just wanted to feel like I was one of the good guys…I was scared that they didn't trust me, so I made sure to show them that I wasn't scared and they could trust me… after that guy (enemy soldier) died, I never wanted to trust anyone ever again…" Mr. Z didn't experience physical losses in this traumatic incident; however, his emotional losses included his plans to make the military his career, his desire to connect with others, and his trust of others. After many years of never sharing about this war-zone event, Mr. Z revealed his need to make a crucial choice to end another's life in order to save his own. While sharing this event in counseling, the veteran grieved, for the first time, the numerous emotional changes within him many years ago from this incident. It was only after he examined in therapy the true impact this event had on his life, as well as tapping into his repressed emotions, that he was able to stop having many of his PTSD symptoms. By expressing profound sadness over his dilemma, Mr. Z was then able to move cognitively and emotionally forward for the first time in over 20 years.

In counseling, the ability to "process" underlying stuck beliefs and emotions by a survivor can have tremendous healing impact because counseling focuses on issues of self-blame, discusses the reality of the details within a traumatic event, addresses distorted beliefs of control, and provides opportunities to fully express grief, loss, and sadness. If one can imagine that a survivor disclosing the details of a traumatic event is, for that person, like sharing his or her most protected and horrifying moment, then one can appreciate the level of trust necessary between counselor and client prior to this information being shared. Providers are encouraged to be open to a wide range of emotional expression, listening closely for statements of self-blame, and handle the information as one would handle a valuable and delicate piece of fine china.

Grief as the root of traumatic stress

Traumatic stress and unresolved grief appear to be highly connected. It is quite possible that the diagnosis of PTSD may also encumber survivors' ability to grieve other situations. Because the symptoms of the disorder may include aspects of chronic grief, the ability to express loss and sadness from either anticipatory grief or more current losses may be limited. Current losses often resonate within a trauma survivor of past losses. Survivors diagnosed with PTSD (with unresolved loss issues as part of their traumatic event) will likely truncate, abbreviate, or deny grieving current losses. Instead, survivors may express alternative emotions or behaviors, such as angry outbursts, a need to control others or having intrusive memories of previous losses. They may express feelings of guilt, depression, or low self-esteem; they may become socially isolated or experience an increase in nightmares.

The nuances of working through unresolved grief and loss vary with each individual survivor or client. In order for those struggling with traumatic stress to begin coping with their losses, a strong rapport is necessary between provider and client. Without a strong trusting relationship, a survivor will often not disclose important information. A thorough assessment regarding a survivor's context currently, as well as during a traumatic event, is also helpful.

An assessment can also include identifying the emotions of guilt, shame, loss, or powerlessness with which the survivor may struggle.

VA SERVICES: A BRIEF SUMMARY

A confusing aspect when attempting to match veteran services and needs of veterans is navigating the diverse resource offerings. VA medical centers (VAMCs) are separate entities from Veteran Benefits (VBA) offices, yet they intersect in terms of what healthcare services veterans are eligible for within VAMCs. VAMCs offer regular hospital or outpatient services for veterans who are eligible, depending on either their military service-connected disability percentage rated by the VBA or their financial means (income), for those who have also served an established minimum of honorable service time. Mental health services are provided at all VAMCs and most Community-based Outpatient Clinics (CBOCs); however some VAMC services will charge a co-pay to veterans who are receiving services which they are not service-connected for or if a veteran is less than 50% service-connected disabled overall. Veterans and providers are encouraged to access the admissions office of their local VAMC or CBOC to learn more about eligibility for VA services. Routing through the process of accessing VA benefits can also include state-level veteran services and the services offered by veteran service organizations (VSOs), such as the American Legion, Veterans of Foreign Wars, and Disabled American Veterans (DAV). This can make the process both beneficial and challenging, as each of these organizations overlaps in some of their offerings, while providing unique services for veterans.

Vet Centers and Readjustment Counseling Service: Grief and bereavement counseling

Grief counseling within Vet Centers and VA medical centers can serve an important role in the recovery for not only those addressing impending death, but also those who have unresolved grief from traumatic events; again, options vary widely. The commonly used phrase, "If you've seen one VA, you've seen one VA," holds true as it applies to grief and bereavement counseling. The best resource to start with is to access the Department of Veterans Affairs website (www.va.gov) in order to locate and identify what exists at a nearby facility. Numerous VA medical facilities do offer hospice and palliative programs, and many include grief groups or counseling.

A multitude of psychotherapy options have been made available over the past 20 years to assist with PTSD within VA facilities and in local communities.

Again, these resources vary, and some may or may not also focus on unresolved grieving. At many VA medical center programs, time-limited, evidence-based treatments are offered to treat PTSD (as well as medication management). Many of the manualized interventions are based on the premise that PTSD is rooted in "obsessive thoughts," although it is the clinical opinion of the author that PTSD may be more complicated than only obsessive thinking about a traumatic incident.

Out in the community are the well-established Vet Centers (formerly known as Veteran Outreach Centers). Vet Centers are part of the Readjustment Counseling Division of VA and have grown from a handful of centers to over 300 over the course of 33 years. Vet Centers specialize in counseling veterans who have served in a war zone, service members or veterans who have survived sexual assault or sexual harassment while in the military, and bereavement cases. Because Vet Centers only work with those meeting the above eligibility criteria, counselors are often adept at identifying symptoms related to unresolved grief and loss, as well as PTSD and other readjustment issues.

Since the advent of the wars in Afghanistan and Iraq, and in collaboration with the Department of Defense (DoD), the Vet Center program provides the first and only established grief counseling by an entire system of the Department of Veterans Affairs. Each of the Vet Centers accepts grief counseling cases after the military reaches out and offers bereavement services to active-duty families. Procedurally, the DoD informs the family about free grief counseling through the Vet Centers. If the family wishes to participate (either individually, as a couple, or as a family), the military will contact the Vet Center regional office serving the geographical area of the family members. The Vet Center regional office then contacts the closest Vet Center in proximity to the family members' residence, and the local Vet Center contacts and offers grief counseling directly to the family. By providing grief counseling to various family members, Vet Centers provide an opportunity for families to maintain their connection with their deceased loved one in a veteran-centric setting. Most grief counseling sessions are provided on an individual basis and allow the family members an opportunity to confidentially discuss the ramifications of the loss of their service member. The eligibility for grief counseling is not limited to war zone deaths, but also includes the death of any active duty service member also recently deceased stateside, and is not time-limited.

CONCLUSION

Grief and loss issues likely have a triggering role for a veteran trauma survivor with PTSD. These situations can include anticipatory grief, since significant losses from the past will potentially be emotionally reactivated as a survivor anticipates the loss of yet another significant relationship. Without counseling or psychotherapy interventions which address unresolved grief, the old patterns of abbreviated grief response will likely be repeated. Part of the goal of effective grief counseling is to provide a safe place where a client can share feelings of vulnerability and horror, as well as fears of past situations. Effective counseling will include a nonjudgmental attitude by the counselor, encouraging a client to express all emotions. Providers can also assist survivors in identifying the many types of losses experienced through a traumatic event. Vet Centers provide bereavement counseling for family members of active-duty service members; VA medical centers have a variety of options, some of which are accessible via hospice and palliative care within the VAMC.

To learn more about Vet Centers, and to locate the closest Vet Center, go to the Vet Center website (www.vetcenter.va.gov).

Lori Daniels, PhD, LCSW, has been involved in the treatment of Posttraumatic Stress Disorder among veterans for over 20 years. She has held positions as director of an outpatient PTSD treatment program with the Honolulu VA Medical Center, as an assistant professor of social work at Hawaii Pacific University in Honolulu, HI, as well as a consultant with the National Center for PTSD - Pacific Islands Division. Daniels is currently the military sexual trauma psychotherapist for the Portland Vet Center and a VA/Hartford geriatric social work scholar.

REFERENCES

Falsetti, S., & Resick, P. (1995). Causal attributions, depression, and post-traumatic stress disorder in victims of crime. *Journal of Applied Social Psychology, 25*, 1027-1042.

Gray, M., & Lombardo, T. (2004). Life event attributions as a potential source of vulnerability following exposure to a traumatic event. *Journal of Loss and Trauma, 9*, 59-72.

Green, B. (2000). Traumatic loss: Conceptual and empirical links between trauma and bereavement. *Journal of Personal and Interpersonal Loss, 5*, 1-17.

Monk, T., Houck, P., & Shear, M. (2006). The daily life of complicated grief patients—what gets missed, what gets added? *Death Studies, 30*(1), 77-85.

Neria, Y., & Litz, B. (2004). Bereavement by traumatic means: The complex synergy of trauma and grief. *Journal of Loss and Trauma, 9,* 73-87.

Raphael, B. (1997). The interaction of trauma and grief. In D. Black, M. Newman, J. Harris-Hendriks, & Mezey, G. (Eds.). *Psychological trauma: A developmental approach* (pp. 31-43). London, England: Gaskell.

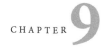

CHAPTER 9

Forgiveness: A Reckoning Process that Facilitates Peace

Deborah Grassman

Combat veterans sometimes come to the end of their lives with unresolved grief or guilt related to military duty. Perhaps this is best captured by a poem entitled *Atoning* by Ron Mann displayed in the National Vietnam Veterans Art Museum in Chicago:

Hoping and wishing
you can settle
this whole thing in your mind
about this war
resolving it within yourself
before the time of atonement comes,
weeping and crying at the end of your life.

Hospice can serve as a last chance to develop peace with unpeaceful memories and to reckon with the guilt of deeds inhumanely committed during war. For some veterans, suppressed memories can no longer be kept at bay. These memories sometimes come forth unbidden because as people come to the end of their lives, their conscious mind gets weaker and their unconscious gets stronger.

Making peace with unpeaceful memories begins by acknowledging guilt that veterans sometimes harbor. Some feel guilty about killing, and this moral injury can sometimes haunt veterans who have not reckoned with it previously. Others feel guilty for *not* killing: "They had to take me off the front lines. I was such a coward."

Noncombat veterans sometimes feel guilty when fellow soldiers volunteer for dangerous missions. One veteran was a talented trumpeter assigned to the Navy band, playing as ships left harbor for Vietnam: "Here I was with this cushy job playing an instrument I loved to play. It wasn't fair." Another veteran said he vicariously sustained trauma with his job handling body bags. "Each of these guys could have been me, except that I was here counting their corpses." Guilt can even sabotage people who were never soldiers at all. One man was sitting at his father's bedside on a hospice unit. The father had served proudly in WWII; the son had been a conscientious objector during the Vietnam War. Later, he became a psychologist and found himself working with Vietnam veterans: "I have a lot of guilt about the impact my actions had on them."

Military nurses and medics can also experience guilt about the life-and-death decisions they made. One nurse said she was not afraid of hell: "I've already been there. I have to live every day with the faces of those soldiers who didn't have a chance during mass casualties. The doctor left it up to me, a 21-year-old nurse, to decide which ones got surgery and which ones were left to die."

Survivor's guilt is common, and it can interfere with veterans' ability to enjoy their lives. One World War II veteran said, "When I landed on the beach, there were all these dead bodies. The sand underneath them was pink with their blood." Then he tearfully added, "They didn't get to have grandkids the way I did." The pleasure he felt with his grandkids was tainted with guilt. "It's not fair that I should have this enjoyment when they can't."

Guilt can also be felt over actions from the war. Some loved the adrenaline rush associated with combat and later have guilt for having enjoyed it. One veteran who had been an especially effective sniper during the Korean War, tearfully lamented his pride in his expertise: "I won many awards for marksmanship, but now I can't believe how much *pride* I took in being able to pick them off. *That's* what hurts the most." Although snipers can be a long way off from their victims, the killing is very graphic because the scope magnifies the target. Others have guilt for killing women and children. Killing enemy soldiers can at least be justified; civilians' deaths cannot, nor can the accidental killing of comrades in what is called "friendly fire." Rumors exist that there were rare instances in which officers who consistently made poor judgments that jeopardized lives of those they commanded were intentionally killed.

Feelings of guilt necessitate the process of forgiveness, and in addition to forgiving themselves, the forgiveness process includes those on the other side: the "enemy." Many veterans have been able to forgive the enemy they fought; others harbor hatred that continues to poison their vitality.

The "enemy" also has to achieve forgiveness. The D-Day Museum in New Orleans has many video clips of veterans among its exhibits. One clip shows a Japanese pilot who had bombed Pearl Harbor. He speaks about how badly he felt for being part of the sneak attack. Such attacks, he says, go against his samurai code; attacks were supposed to be out in the open so they could be fair. In the next scene, this same pilot meets with one of the Pearl Harbor survivors. They talk about forgiveness. The Japanese veteran leaves a rose at the Pearl Harbor Memorial to honor the soldiers, sailors, and marines he had killed, acknowledging his remorse. Now he sends the American veteran money to leave a rose at the memorial annually.

Some Vietnam veterans struggle with forgiving the government for how they feel they were used and betrayed. Korean and Vietnam veterans might have to forgive the American public for ignoring or scorning them. Forgiveness is not just between people either. Soldiers have to forgive the world for being unfair and for having cruelty and war in it; they have to forgive God for allowing the world to be a world with war in it.

Jim, a World War II veteran, was at a VA Medical Center. Weak with a cancer that would take his life in a few days, he was seen by Deborah, a hospice and palliative care nurse practitioner consultant. She spoke to him quietly for several minutes about hospice care, and then inquired if there was anything from the war that might still be troubling him. Jim said there was, but he was too ashamed to say it out loud. Motioning for Deborah to come down close to him, he whispered, "Do you have any idea how many men I've killed?"

Deborah shook her head, remaining silent, steadily meeting his gaze with her own. He continued.

"Do you have any idea how many throats I've slit?"

Again she shook her head. The image was grim, and Deborah felt her eyes begin to tear. Jim was tearful too. They sat silently together, sharing Jim's suffering. No words needed to be said. This was a sacred moment that words would only corrupt.

After several minutes, Deborah asked, "Would it be meaningful if I said a prayer asking for forgiveness?"

He nodded. Deborah placed her hand on Jim's chest, anchoring his flighty, anxious energy with the security of her relaxed palm (Simpson, 1999). Her prayer, like any praying she does with veterans, reflected no particular religion. "Dear God: This man comes before you acknowledging the pain he has caused others. He has killed; he has maimed. He hurts with the pain of knowing what he did. He hurts with the pain of humanity. He comes before you now asking for forgiveness. He needs your mercy to restore his integrity. He comes before you saying, 'Forgive me for the wrongs I have committed.' Dear God, help him feel your saving grace. Restore this man to wholeness so he can come home to you soon. Amen."

Jim kept his eyes closed for a moment, tears streaming down from unopened lids. Then he opened his eyes and smiled gratefully; his new sense of peace was almost palpable. It was a reminder of just how heavy guilt weighs, and the importance of acknowledging the need for forgiveness.

CREATING SAFE EMOTIONAL ENVIRONMENTS THAT FACILITATE FORGIVENESS

Experiencing or witnessing violence can be disturbing for anyone; the difference with veterans is that they committed much of the violence. That is a deeper level of traumatization. Guilt and shame can manifest itself in the final days of life. While this may only occur in a small percentage of dying veterans, it can greatly complicate peaceful dying because it can cause anguish and agitation. Forgiveness can bring peace with this kind of painful past. Although the past cannot be changed, the *relationship* to the past can. Forgiveness is the means to that end.

The dictionary (Webster, 1995) defines the word forgive as "to give up resentment against or the desire to punish." This punishment might include self-punishment. It is the inability to forgive one's self for letting others die or, worse, for killing others, that keeps some veterans in darkness; shame seals light from their souls. It is this moral injury that soldiers sustained that sometimes surfaces as they lie in a hospice bed facing their own deaths.

One crucial component of self-forgiveness is learning to distinguish guilt from shame. Guilt is natural and designed to provide feedback so important lessons can be learned; shame is artificially created and designed to punish. Guilt tells us something we *did* is wrong, guiding us toward more compassionate actions of others. Shame tells us that *we* are wrong, filling us with worthlessness and negating self-compassion. Guilt mobilizes people into new behaviors; shame causes immobilization. Veterans are sometimes filled with shame. They need to go from shame to guilt so they can get to forgiveness.

Forgiveness can, unknowingly, be faked. A veteran might say, "I let that go a long time ago" or "It's over and forgotten." Sometimes, that is true. At other times, it is a way to avoid the work of forgiveness. Assessment is needed to make the distinction.

It is essential that clinicians know how to create a safe emotional environment that invites the veteran to consider forgiveness. However, this needs to be done carefully and cautiously. At no time should the clinician overtly, covertly, or subtly convey to the veteran that he "needs to forgive." This can actually add another layer of damage by causing the veteran to feel additional guilt about not being able to achieve forgiveness. Rather, the clinician should simply offer the consideration of forgiveness and invite the veteran to stay open to its possibility.

Bearing witness to a veteran's story can begin the healing process. Honoring veterans for their service to their country is a simple act that often precipitates the story-telling process. There are many ways to honor veterans. Ceremonially pinning veterans with an American flag pin or presenting them with a military certificate that cites their service and displays the seal of their branch of service are simple, yet effective ways. The team schedules a ceremony with the family and may even videotape the ceremony to preserve the memory. Veterans who are institutionalized in a facility might be ceremonially presented with an American flag that is then placed on their door, notifying all who enter of the military service that has been rendered. Flags, certificates, and pins offer cues for any staff walking into the environment. These cues can act as prompts for the clinician to acknowledge military service and express gratitude, which then often precipitates military stories from the veteran.

Memorial monuments can be a catalyst for military stories. Honor Flight is a program that flies World War II veterans to see the WWII memorial in Washington, D.C. Visiting memorial monuments is important because the monuments often serve as a repository for shame, precipitating the courage to seek forgiveness. The Honor Flight program plans to begin flights for Korea and Vietnam veterans as well.

Therapeutic letter writing can be very effective to help facilitate healing and forgiveness (Grassman, 2012). For example, a photo of a young Vietnamese father and his daughter was left at the Vietnam Veterans Memorial (Jaffe, 2005). This note was attached to the photo:

> *Dear Sir, for 22 years I have carried your picture in my wallet. I was only 18 years old that day we faced one another...Why you didn't take my life I'll never know. You stared at me so long, armed with your AK-47, and yet you did not fire. Forgive me for taking your life. So many times over the years I have stared at your picture and your daughter, I suspect. Each time my heart and guts would burn with the pain of guilt...Forgive me, Sir.*

This man achieved forgiveness *before* he came to the end of his life. Yet his story, and others like his, can reveal dark acts that the veteran shielded from other peoples' awareness or even their own. Veterans often respond to an inquiry about unfinished business from their wartime experience: "Is there anything from your military service that might still be troubling you now?" This question might elicit stories that had previously been locked behind a facade. After the story is told, it is not unusual for a family member to comment, "I've never heard that story before. I had no idea."

When asking this kind of question, it is important to allow time and space for the answer to emerge. It is also important to not make veterans feel pressured to answer the question at all or to feel judged if they decline. Clinician pressure or judgment can be conveyed nonverbally; small inflections in the voice or subtle body language can communicate the clinician's agenda. To guard against this, clinicians should practice self-monitoring techniques, as well as invite feedback from colleagues. If clinicians are unaware or are disconnected from personal hostility they express in everyday life, they will have a difficult time understanding the hostilities committed by the veteran. The veteran, consciously or unconsciously, will sense this, feel judged, and not disclose. If clinicians justify their own misdeeds, they will tend to do the same with the veteran, bypassing important opportunities to precipitate healing.

For example, it is important to not try to minimize a veteran's guilt or soothe it with rationalizations: "That was a long time ago" or "You were just obeying orders." These types of clinician responses essentially say to the veteran: "Don't tell me about your guilt and shame. Put it back behind that stoic wall." Veterans know when and why they killed, and whether or not it violates their deepest-held moral beliefs. What they need is to have the guilt acknowledged and accepted so they can finally forgive themselves.

Not all staff members can be expected to be facilitators of forgiveness. Many agencies have developed teams of chaplains and social workers who specialize in responding to these situations. All staff need to know how to initially respond to issues of guilt and shame; they can then make a referral to specialized team members who can follow up with assessment and intervention.

If the veteran becomes agitated with wartime memories, especially if he is in the last several days of life, the "hand-heart connection" can support emotional safety (Simpson, 1999). In this technique, the clinician places his or her hand firmly on the veteran's chest. This gesture is usually very calming for the veteran because anxious energy usually rises; the voice gets higher pitched and energy gets flighty. A calm, centered person's energy usually resides lower and deeper. If a calm person places his or her hand on an unsettled person's sternum, it can often help the anxious person to feel secure, more stable, less anxious, and safe to feel whatever they are experiencing. This securing gesture is often practiced unconsciously when people get excited, and they will place their palm over their own sternum to anchor themselves. Family members can be taught to do the hand-heart connection with the veteran. It not only helps the agitated veteran, it often helps family members with their own sense of helplessness.

THE CLINICIAN'S ROLE IN FACILITATING FORGIVENESS: A SUMMARY

A few simple tenets related to forgiveness can provide a foundation for clinicians so that forgiveness is more likely to be achieved:

- Acknowledge the veteran's military service. Express gratitude.
- Offer the possibility that there may be troubling military issues that could be an understandable source of distress.
- Do not dismiss or minimize guilt with well-intentioned platitudes. Instead, create a safe emotional environment so that guilt and shame can be revealed if the veteran so chooses.
- Do not push veterans into forgiveness; this only causes further damage. Instead, invite them to stay open to its possibility.
- Practice self-awareness about personal hostility. Otherwise, clinicians will have a difficult time understanding the hostilities committed by the veteran. The veteran, consciously or unconsciously, will sense this, feel judged, and not disclose.
- If the veteran is agitated with wartime memories, teach the veteran's family how to do the hand-heart connection.
- Make a referral to team members who specialize in forgiveness.

Deborah Grassman, ARNP, is a nurse practitioner. Her career at Bay Pines VA in St. Petersburg, FL, lasted for nearly 30 years, where she was the director of the hospice program. She recently retired from the VA and now provides education and consultation throughout the country. Ms. Grassman is the author of Peace at Last: Stories of Hope and Healing for Veterans and Their Families *(Vandamere Press, 2009) and* The Hero Within: Redeeming the Destiny We Were Born to Fulfill *(Vandamere Press, 2012).*

REFERENCES

Grassman, D. (2009). *Peace at last: Stories of hope and healing for veterans and their families*. St. Petersburg, FL: Vandamere Press.

Grassman, D. (2012). *The hero within: Redeeming the destiny we were born to fulfill*. St. Petersburg, FL: Vandamere Press.

Jaffe, G. (2005, August 17). War wounds. *The Wall Street Journal*.

Neufeldt, V., & Sparks, A. (Eds.). (1995). *Webster's new world dictionary*. New York, NY: Simon & Schuster, Inc.

Simpson, M. (1999). Therapeutic touch: For those who accompany the dying. In S. Bertman (Ed.), *Grief and the Healing Arts*. Amityville, NY: Baywood.

CHAPTER 10

Voices
A Voice From a Clinician

Deborah Grassman

I nside most stoical patients is a gentle, sensitive human being just waiting for a chance to emerge. The reality that many of these veterans committed violent acts does not mean that these veterans had no tenderness in them. Tenderness breeds compassion; that compassion must be covered up with a hardened shell in order to fight and kill. Unfortunately, the shell might remain when the war is done. Sometimes guilt or horror over what they have seen or done seals the shell, but this guilt often needs to be faced and felt so the soldiers can heal and come home to themselves.

Guilt weighed heavily on Barry, a World War II veteran who lived at the Ohio State Veterans Home. Stein Hospice provides end-of-life care at the facility, and Stein Hospice staff asked me to train them in how to better care for dying veterans. They wanted me to meet with Barry because he had aggressive and combative behaviors. I met with the 92-year-old veteran, along with 10 hospice staff who were observing the interaction. Staff had given Barry my book, *Peace at Last: Stories of Hope and Healing for Veterans and Their Families* (2009), and he was eager to meet me.

Initially, Barry and I talked about his relationship with his three estranged sons and his anger at being confined to a nursing home. Then, I asked him about his military service.

"Wanna hear about my three Purple Hearts and two Bronze Stars?" he asked me proudly.

"No. We can talk about your medals later," I said gently. "Right now I'd be interested in hearing about things from World War II that might still be troubling you."

Barry's pride quickly turned to hostility. "All of it!" he said fiercely, wheeling quickly around to bring his face close to mine. I said nothing, but my eyes opened in surprise, and I motioned for him to proceed.

"Do you know what it's like to put a gun in the middle of a forehead and pull the trigger?" he asked intently, putting his forefinger in the middle of my forehead, pushing my head back.

Even though I had heard these kinds of stories from other veterans, I was unprepared for the intensity and fierceness with which he had responded. I summoned inner strength so that I could remain steadfast. My eyes never diverted from his. I shook my head "no," acknowledging that I did not know what that was like.

"Ya wanna hear more?" he asked in a taunting manner.

I did not indicate yes or no. I simply remained open to the anger and bitterness he was directing toward me.

He paused before he proceeded. "Do you know what it's like to tie a noose around a man's neck and watch him hang?" He leaned forward peering even more intently at me.

Again, I met his steely blue eyes that were piercing my soul with a steady gaze that belied the inner quaking I was experiencing as I imagined the horror that he had seen and done.

"Wanna hear more of what I did?" he challenged me.

Again, I said nothing, but my unwavering gaze let him know I could take it.

Barry then retracted his stance slightly and told me that he and a buddy had been ordered to patrol an occupied city. The names of the occupants were posted on the doors of the houses. They had gone into one house, however, and found three teenage boys whose names were not on the list.

"They weren't supposed to be there. They were just lying on their beds jeering at us with their arms behind their heads." Barry put his arms behind his head to show me how the boys looked. "The other soldier I was with asked me what we should do with 'em. I told him that we gotta peel 'em."

I narrowed my eyes quizzically, indicating that I did not know what he meant.

Barry came close to my face, pushing back the bill of his Army hat so he could get even closer. "You split their heads open with the bullet. Their brains come out."

Tears came to my eyes as I imagined the shockingly intimate carnage.

"Yeah. Ya see? Want to hear more *NOW*?"

I shook my head no. "I can't hear any more," I told him without averting my gaze from his. "I've heard all I can hear."

Seconds ticked by as we sat locked together in silent wartime memories. The room was reeling, and I was not sure what to do next. Instinctively, I did the hand-heart connection, placing my hand firmly on his heart while my eyes peered closely into his soul, a place beyond the anger and venom he was spewing forth. "Barry, I am so sorry that you were put in a position to see and do the things that you had to see and do at that young, tender age. I am so sorry that you had to experience that."

I felt Barry relax under my hand. Then tears came to his eyes, and we cried together. "I'm shaking," he said.

"That's okay, Barry. Let yourself shake, just breathe deeply as you shake. Breathe and shake and cry."

Barry had great trust in the chaplain, so I motioned for Chaplain Vern to stand behind Barry and encircle him in a hug that could contain the trembling. I motioned for the other staff to draw in closely as well.

"Barry. We're here to encircle you with love while Chaplain Vern prays for you. Is that okay with you?"

Barry indicated consent, and Chaplain Vern prayed for peace in Barry's soul. Barry continued to cry and shake, even making low guttural noises. Afterward, he looked up with amazement at the team surrounding him, a team who had the courage to bear witness to his story. A look of relief came over Barry's face. Softness crept in to replace his furled and fierce brow.

Marie, a Vietnam War veteran who is one of my colleagues and had traveled with me, came forward. "Barry, I have a pin I want to honor you with." Marie showed him an American flag pin inscribed with "honored veteran." Barry remained silent, but held his gaze into Marie's eyes. "You deserve this. You have carried the guilt long enough. It took a lot of courage to do what you did here today. I want you to have this." Marie pinned his shirt collar and then enveloped him in a hug. Once again, Barry cried. In fact, all of us did. We were witnessing a soldier brought home from war at last.

Barry maintained his softness for the many months he lived. He was smiling, and even seemed light-hearted. He reconciled with two of his sons. Staff members were astounded with the change in him; I was not surprised by the change. Combat is like that. It can create mean and ugly places in veterans' souls, and those places can be covered up during much of a person's life. At the end of life, however, redemption awaits if veterans have the courage to avail themselves of the opportunity the way Barry did, and clinicians have the courage to learn how to create safe emotional environments so the story can emerge if the veteran so chooses.

Deborah Grassman, *ARNP, is a nurse practitioner. Her career at Bay Pines VA in St. Petersburg, FL, lasted for nearly 30 years, where she was the director of the hospice program. She recently retired from the VA and now provides education and consultation throughout the country. Ms. Grassman is the author of* Peace at Last: Stories of Hope and Healing for Veterans and Their Families *(Vandamere Press, 2009) and* The Hero Within: Redeeming the Destiny We Were Born to Fulfill *(Vandamere Press, 2012).*

CHAPTER 11

Special Issues in Pain Management

V.S. Periyakoil

The prevalence of chronic pain in the adult population ranges from 2% to 40%, with a median point prevalence of 15% (Manchikanti, 2006). Pain affects more than 50% of older persons living in a community setting and more than 80% of nursing home residents. Persistent pain is widely prevalent in veterans with serious illnesses and is often underdiagnosed and ineffectively managed. Pain limits functional status and can result in diminished quality of life, sleep disturbances, social isolation, depression, and increased healthcare costs and resource utilization.

Timely and effective assessment and judicious management of pain in veterans will help in alleviating their suffering, while maintaining and augmenting quality of life.

TERMS COMMONLY USED WHEN DESCRIBING PHYSICAL PAIN

- *Nociceptive pain* is the perception of nociceptive input, usually due to tissue damage (e.g., postoperative pain). Nociceptive pain is further subdivided into somatic and visceral pain. *Somatic pain* is pain arising from injury to body tissues. It is well localized but variable in description and experience. *Visceral pain* is pain arising from the viscera mediated by stretch receptors. It is poorly localized, deep, dull, and cramping (e.g., pain associated with appendicitis, hepatic cancer metastasis, bowel ischemia).
- *Neuropathic pain* is pain initiated or caused by a primary lesion or dysfunction in the nervous system.
- *Central pain* is pain initiated or caused by a primary lesion or dysfunction in the central nervous system (e.g. post-stroke pain, phantom limb pain).
- *Wind-up pain* is the slow temporal summation of pain mediated by C fibers of repetitive noxious stimulation at a rate less than one stimulus per 3 seconds. It may cause the person to experience a gradual increase in the perceived magnitude of pain.

PAIN ASSESSMENT

Pain presentation in veterans may be skewed due to a variety of factors including the culture of stoicism and battlemind as well as due to co-morbid conditions like depression, Posttraumatic Stress Disorder (PTSD), and recreational substance usage. A thorough assessment is necessary to formulate a plan to successfully treat persistent pain. The International Association for the Study of Pain (IASP) has developed taxonomy for the classification of pain that identifies five axes as below and these are a helpful framework in assessing pain.

- *Axis I: Anatomic regions*: Ask patient to point out specific areas in the body where they have pain.
- *Axis II: Organ systems*: Identify possible organs that may be involved. It is important to remember areas of referred pain, e.g. diaphragmatic pain to shoulder.
- *Axis III: Temporal characteristics, pattern of occurrence*: Assess the time the pain occurs, and exacerbating and relieving factors.
- *Axis IV: Intensity, time since onset of pain*: Some older adults may be able to use numbers (scale of 0 to 10) to describe intensity while other may prefer words (mild, moderate and severe).
- *Axis V: Etiology*: Underlying etiology of pain should be identified and reversible problems should be corrected.

Pain assessment should include an exploration of effects of pain on functional status, sleep, libido, emotional and social well-being. Scales such as the McGill Pain Questionnaire and the Pain Disability Scale measure pain in a variety of domains, including the intensity, location, and affect. Although time-intensive, scales measuring multiple domains can provide a wealth of information about the patient's unique experience of pain. It is also prudent to concurrently screen for PTSD and depression. When patients are unable or unwilling to cooperate with time-intensive pain assessments, simple scales like the Numeric Rating Scale and the Faces Pain Scale are effective. The patient is asked to rate his or her pain by assigning a numerical value (with 0 indicating no pain and 10 representing the worst pain imaginable), or a facial expression corresponding to the pain.

The persistent pain experience in veterans is often influenced by certain unique factors that are common in veterans. Military service exposes men and women in service to specific training and common life experiences and stressors that shape their thinking, behaviors, and experiences. Three types of stress are common in Americans who serve in the armed services and these may influence how they experience and interpret disease-related pain.

a. *Life threat*: This is a prevalent issue in combat veterans and prisoners of war.

b. *Loss of colleagues and friends, loss of relationships and loss of limbs in the line of duty*: The loss of functionality often seen with persistent pain and the losses inherent in the chronic and serious illness process may remind veterans of past losses when they were on service, when their friends and "buddies" died in front of their eyes, or even in their arms, in combat. Loss of limbs and shrapnel injuries may trigger unusual pain syndromes like phantom pain and other neuropathic pain syndromes.

c. *Inner conflict*: During active duty, men and women in service may be forced to carry out actions that may be in conflict with their fundamental values and beliefs. For example, they may have to kill enemy soldiers or may inadvertently harm civilians and women and children in the line of duty. This may be at odds with their personal values of being compassionate or not hurting others. Also, the presence of ongoing challenging circumstances during a tour of duty may take a toll on their physical and emotional health. These experiences will skew how they experience and interpret pain due to serious illness. For example, a veteran who killed an enemy soldier in the line of duty may feel tremendous guilt and moral distress as she or he is now wrestling with a life-limiting illness and doing a life review as a part of the dying process. Depending on their spiritual and religious beliefs, they may have worries about life after death and if and how that may be influenced by their past actions in the line of duty.

THE VETERAN CULTURE, BATTLEMIND TRAINING, AND STOICISM

Culture consists of the beliefs, behaviors, objects, and other characteristics common to the members of a particular group; in this case, members of the armed forces. Battlemind is defined as a soldier's inner strength to face fear and adversity during combat, with courage. It is the will to persevere and win. When on a tour of duty, a person is expected to be strong and fully operational at all times. There is a strong stigma associated with any show of weakness. They cannot back away from the warfront. They are expected to meet challenges head on, and maintain mental toughness during times of adversity and challenge. For example, the United States Navy Sea Air and Land (SEAL) personnel often quote the phrase, "the only easy day was yesterday." This battlemind mindset, which comes from the ongoing rigorous training they receive when on active duty, often becomes an integral part of who they are. When faced with physical threats due to serious illness, veterans often work hard to meet the illness-related challenges with courage and stoicism. Data show that veterans, as a cultural group, are at a higher risk for PTSD, depression, and substance abuse. The cluster of these experiences will likely influence how pain is experienced and interpreted. In a recent study (Tan, Teo, Anderson, and Jensen, 2011) of pain and coping conducted on a group of 109 veterans with chronic pain, researchers studied nine specific pain-related adaptive and maladaptive coping and belief domains: guarding, exercise/stretch, resting, catastrophizing, control, disability, harm, medication, and pacing. Each of the nine pain-related coping responses and beliefs were classified as adaptive (exercise/stretch, control, and pacing) or maladaptive (guarding, resting, catastrophizing, disability, harm, and medication). The study results showed that maladaptive coping and beliefs play a more powerful role than adaptive coping and beliefs in predicting pain interference and depression and that adaptive responses may be more important than maladaptive responses in predicting reported pain intensity.

Posttraumatic Stress Disorder (PTSD) and pain in veterans

An estimated 25% (Breslau, Davis, Andreski, and Peterson, 1991) who have been exposed to trauma go on to develop Posttraumatic Stress Disorder (PTSD) during their lifetime. PTSD is also more common in war veterans with an estimated prevalence of about 30% in Vietnam veterans, about 10% of the Gulf War (Desert Storm) veterans, about 6% to 11% of the Afghanistan war veterans, and about 12% to 20% of the Iraq war veterans (Boscarino, 2008). Hispanic veterans are said to exhibit higher risk of developing PTSD than veterans of other racial/ethnic backgrounds. Possible mediators of the effects of Hispanic ethnicity on vulnerability to PTSD are identified, including psychosocial factors (racial/ethnic discrimination and alienation) and sociocultural influences (stoicism and normalization of stress alexithymia and fatalism). PTSD is associated with chronic pain syndromes. PTSD is also associated with poor coping skills and can thus amplify the distress or lead to refractory pain and non-pain symptoms. Many seriously ill patients suffer from symptoms like pain, dyspnea, nausea, fatigue and many others and these could be exacerbated by PTSD. A key fact in terms of how PTSD influences the pain experience is that trauma-related memory can be triggered by somatosensory triggers.

For example, cancer pain may trigger repeated flashbacks for a PTSD patient who was tortured in a concentration camp when he was a prisoner of war. Additionally, avoidance symptoms are central to the diagnosis of PTSD; these patients tend to cope by avoiding or ignoring problems (Amir et al., 1997; Bryant and Harvey, 1995). In some cases, patients may use maladaptive coping strategies like alcohol or recreational drugs to cope with pain that may be a manifestation of a serious illness like cancer or coronary arterial disease. This may cause a delay in the diagnosis of the underlying illness and result in increased mortality and morbidity in these patients.

The interaction between PTSD and pain

When PTSD patients start experiencing pain as a part of their serious illness process, the following issues need to be considered.

a. Patients with even remote history of recreational opioid usage often have high tolerance to opioids and will likely need higher doses of opioids to control their illness-related pain. These patients are also more prone to refractory pain syndromes and require skilled palliative care services. Due to their past experiences with recreational drugs, they may be very knowledgeable about opioids and may tend to self-manage their medications and not adhere entirely to the regimens prescribed.

b. Some patients may exhibit "pseudoaddictive behavior" due to poorly controlled pain. "Pseudoaddiction" is a phenomenon that occurs when a patient who is suffering with a legitimate chronic pain condition is undertreated with pain medication (Weissman, 2006). The situation arises when the clinician is reluctant to provide enough medication to assure adequate symptom relief for a patient who requires a higher dose of long-acting (basal) pain medication. This can provoke a series of "conditioned behaviors" focused on acquisition of the controlled drug that can appear to indicate aberrant addictive-type behaviors. To note, some patients may even revert back to taking street drugs to supplement their inadequate pain medications and this causes tremendous angst in patients and their families as they slip back into dysfunctional old patterns of behavior. For example, the patient may become furtive and avoidant and family members may start policing his or her activities. As all parties are aware that the patient is seriously ill, they may feel significant guilt. Patients also feel intense preparatory grief in addition to being at risk for depression (Periyakoil, 2012). In pseudoaddiction, the behaviors tend to disappear when an adequate amount of the drug is prescribed. It behooves clinicians to carefully consider what opioids to use in these patients. Methadone is an effective choice for basal pain control. Newer drugs like suboxone are also effective when there are compelling concerns about abuse.

c. The need for pain medications and the dependence on clinicians for care plan management may undermine the patient's sense of control and thereby create a sense of hostility or non-compliance in the patient and undermine the therapeutic relationship. Frank and ongoing discussions are vitally important in engaging the patient in an ongoing manner.

Prescription drug abuse: Non-medical use of prescription drugs is the second most prevalent category of drug abuse, after marijuana. The risk for abuse or dependence was highest for prescribed psychoactive drugs (Chassen et al., 2001). The most commonly abused opioid class of drugs (Manchikanti, 2006) include oxycodone (Percodan, Percocet, Roxicet, Tylox, OxyContin), hydrocodone (Vicodin, Vicoprofen, Lorcet, Lortab), hydromorphone, methadone, morphine (Astramorph, Duramorph, MS Contin, Roxanol), and codeine. Data from Department of Health and Human Services (DHHS, 2002, 2004, 2006) and Substance Abuse and Mental Health Services Administration (SAMHSA, 2004) show that while opioids are by far the most abused drugs, other controlled substances such as benzodiazepines, sedative hypnotics, and central nervous system stimulants, though described as having less potential for abuse, are also of major concern as they appear to be widely used for non-medical purposes as well. Substance abuse often coexists with PTSD (Chilcoat and Breslau, 1998; Deykin and Buka, 1997; Jacobsen, Southwick, and Kosten, 2001; Saxon et al., 2001) with PTSD patients being at more than a fourfold risk for misuse and dependence. Data suggest that drug abuse or dependence in persons with PTSD might be caused by efforts to self-medicate. It is very important to routinely screen all patients for PTSD before prescribing opioids. If they screen positive for PTSD, they should be immediately referred to a mental health professional for further evaluation. In veterans with mental health issues, analgesic regimens should ideally be charted with ongoing input from the patient, their primary family member(s), the primary care provider and mental health professional. Constant education about appropriate adherence to opioid regimen is vital to minimize misuse, abuse, diversion, or concurrent recreational drug use.

TREATMENT

Approaches to persistent pain treatment

All patients should be educated about their persistent pain, the underlying causes, and how best to track its location, intensity, and how to take medications properly. They should be encouraged to use non-pharmacological modalities and exercise regularly. They should be educated about availability of support groups and other VA services based on their specific needs (PTSD support groups, Alcoholics Anonymous, Narcotics Anonymous). Family members of veterans should be educated as well about the patient's illness condition. The more we are able to empower veterans and families to take a central role in their illness management, the better will be their outcomes.

Nonpharmacologic therapy

Recognizing the common overlap of depression, anxiety, and PTSD should prompt early consultation with mental health professionals. Psychological interventions and cognitive-behavioral therapy (CBT) are also important tools for treatment of persistent pain as they help patients cope with the stresses that accompany persistent pain. In CBT, patients are asked to track their pain and record the thoughts that are associated with the pain experience to identify maladaptive coping strategies, including misuse of prescription medications, alcohol, or recreational substance use. By conscientiously replacing these maladaptive strategies with positive coping strategies, patients can increase control over pain-related experiences and thereby over the pain. When possible, family members and caregivers should be included in the care planning and even in the therapy.

The importance of exercise cannot be overstated. Exercise (to the extent the patient can tolerate it) will maintain functional status, boost mood, and promote a sense of independence and control. For patients who are unable to tolerate weight-bearing exercises due to osteoarthritis, metastatic bone disease, etc., pool therapy (which is available in many VA facilities) should be offered. For patients with advanced illness who are bed-bound, gentle passive range of motion exercises and massage therapy are effective. The goals of therapy should be determined after discussion with the veteran (or the surrogate decision maker in cognitively-impaired patients). Such goals may include optimizing quality of life, improving functional status, minimizing dependence on prescription medications, and maintaining abstinence from nicotine, alcohol, or recreational drugs.

An interdisciplinary team approach to treatment may be strongly recommended for patients with complex pain. Including occupational therapists, physical therapists, massage therapists, mental health experts and the chaplain should be considered on a case-by-case basis. Incorporating complementary and alternative modalities such as hypnosis, aromatherapy, biofeedback, music, and pet therapy are especially valuable as they have minimal to no side effects.

Pharmacologic therapy

When starting pharmacologic therapy, nonsystemic therapies should be tried first. For example, patients that primarily have knee pain might respond to intra-articular corticosteroid injections. Topical preparations such as capsaicin or diclofenac gel or lidocaine patches might be effective. If these local therapies are ineffective, systemic therapy should be instituted and the patient should be educated to ensure understanding of the need to take medications as prescribed. The pain ladder from the World Health Organization (WHO) offers a globally-accepted approach towards analgesic management. Using relatively innocuous medications like acetaminophen for many mild to moderate pain syndromes, particularly osteoarthritic pain, is recommended as first-line therapy. The maximum adult dose is 4gm/day and in an older adult population the recommendation is to adhere to a maximum dosage of 3gm /d. For patients at risk of liver dysfunction, particularly those who have a history of alcohol intake, the dosage should be decreased by 50%, or acetaminophen should be avoided. Acetaminophen administration frequency should be based on the patient's renal function. For patients with a Creatinine clearance of 10-50 mL/minute it can be dosed every six hours and for patients with a Creatinine clearance of <10 mL/minute it should be given every eight hours. Non-Steroidal Anti-Inflammatory Drugs (NSAIDs) are effective for chronic inflammatory pain and are used after acetaminophen has been tried and proven to be ineffective. NSAID side effects include renal dysfunction, GI bleeding, platelet dysfunction, and fluid retention; due to these significant adverse effects, they are better limited for short-term use, especially in older adults (O'Neil, Hanlon, and Marcum, 2012). Patients with history of ulcer disease or complication, those who are on dual antiplatelet therapy, or are on an NSAID with concomitant anticoagulant therapy are at high risk for GI toxicity (2008 American College of Cardiology Foundation/ American College of Gastroenterology (ACG)/American Heart Association guidelines). Additional risk factors for NSAID GI toxicity include age ≥60 years, corticosteroid use, dyspepsia or GERD symptoms. Topical NSAIDs appear to be safe and effective in the short term, but longer-term studies are lacking.

Moderate to severe pain or pain that requires chronic treatment often requires opioid medications for sufficient relief, though the evidence base supporting the role of long-term opioids in persistent non-cancer pain is sparse. Common adverse events included constipation (median frequency of occurrence = 30%), nausea (28%), dizziness (22%), and prompted opioid discontinuation in 25% of cases. Careful and ongoing monitoring for benefits and side effects and tailoring therapy to the individual patient's response to the therapeutic regimen are keys to successful treatment.

In general, continuous and persistent pain due to a serious illness should be treated with long-acting or sustained-release formulations after opioid requirements have been estimated by an initial trial of a short-acting agent. Breakthrough pain is to be treated with rapidly acting medications with short half-lives. A typical patient requires approximately 5% to 15% of the total daily dose offered approximately every 4 hours orally for breakthrough pain. The drug dose and dosing intervals should be varied based on the patient's liver and kidney function. Tolerance develops fairly rapidly to other adverse events of opioids, such as respiratory depression and sedation; constipation usually accompanies opioid use as the opioids bind to the mu receptors found in the gut and slow down peristalsis. In fact, the most common adverse event of opioid treatment is constipation, and tolerance to constipation does not occur. Experts recommend starting therapy with a stimulant laxative (such as sienna) concurrently with the opioid unless the patient has signs or symptoms of bowel obstruction. Respiratory depression is the most serious potential adverse effect associated with opioid use, but tolerance to this effect develops quickly. Older adults with a history of lung dysfunction are at particular risk when opioid dosages are increased too rapidly or when a benzodiazepine is prescribed concomitantly. It is important to educate patients about the risks of increased falls and instruct them not to drive or operate heavy equipment when opioids are started or the dosage changed. (Please see Tables 1 and 2 for further resources on principles of using opioids in persistent pain management.)

Adjuvant medications can be used effectively solely or in combination with opioids for treating patients with neuropathic pain or mixed pain syndromes. Tricyclic antidepressants (TCAs) are effective in the treatment of post-herpetic neuralgia and diabetic neuropathy. Clinical depression in patients with persistent pain requires treatment to achieve optimal analgesia and quality of life and selective serotonin re-uptake inhibitors (SSRIs) are the first-line class of drugs. Duloxetine, an inhibitor of norepinephrine and serotonin uptake, is approved both as an antidepressant and for the treatment of pain from diabetic neuropathy and may offer a more favorable adverse-event profile than the TCAs.

Adverse effects of opioids in some veterans with PTSD

PTSD patients use dissociation to cope with their resurgent traumatic memories. Some terminally-ill patients who are on narcotic analgesics or sedative hypnotics for palliation of their disease-related symptoms are unable to dissociate from their trauma-related memories which now seep through into their conscious mind. Thus, the opioids and benzodiazepines can precipitate distressing flashbacks and nightmares in these patients. In such cases, some patients who find the intrusive symptoms extremely distressing refuse to take opioid pain medication even in the face of severe pain due to the terminal illness; they prefer to endure the physical pain due to the terminal illness over dealing with the PTSD-related emotional pain that may be precipitated by the mind-altering property of the opioids and psychotropic medications. This may be distressing to the family and to the healthcare team as they have to witness the patient's physical pain but are unable to palliate it with opioids. However, it is critical in these situations to empower the patient and respect their decision to forego opioids and other psychotropic medications and palliate their symptoms using non-pharmacological therapeutic modalities like support groups, trauma-focused group therapy (Schnurr et al., 2003), massage therapy, music therapy, and relaxation therapy. Specific modalities like eye movement desensitization and reprocessing (Taylor, 2003) are more feasible for palliative care patients with an anticipated life-span of months to years.

In conclusion, careful and thorough assessment of pain in all seriously ill veterans requires a comprehensive approach that includes bio-psycho-socio-spiritual aspects and also carefully considers the culture of veterans and how that may affect their perception and interpretation of their pain. Effective management of pain will prevent erosion and conserve and augment (Periyakoil, 2012) dignity for all seriously ill veterans.

How to institute opioid therapy (Table 1)

When dosing opioids for a patient with chronic severe pain remember the following:

by mouth	(When giving pain medications, the oral route is always preferred over other routes like transdermal, intravenous or sub-cutaneous routes)
by the clock	(Chronic basal pain is usually best treated with scheduled long acting pain medications, with short acting pain medications on an as-needed basis for incidental or break through pain)
by the ladder	Pain Ladder from the World Health Organization

Opioid Equivalency Table (Table 2)

Drug	Oral/Rectal Route	Parenteral Route	Conversion Ratio to Oral Morphine	Equianalgesic Dose of Oral Morphine
Morphine sulfate	30mg Oral morphine	10mg of parenteral morphine	Parenteral morphine is **3 times** as potent as oral morphine	30mg Oral morphine
Oxycodone	20mg of oral oxycodone	N/A	Oral Oxycodone is **roughly 1.5 times** more potent than oral morphine	30mg Oral morphine
Hydrocodone	20mg of oral hydrocodone	N/A	Oral hydrocodone is **roughly 1.5 times** more potent than oral morphine	30mg Oral morphine
Hydromorphone	7mg of oral hydromorphone	1.5mg of parenteral hydromorphone	Oral hydromorphone is about **4-7 times** as potent as oral morphine Parenteral hydromorphone is **20 times** as potent as oral morphine	30mg Oral morphine
Fentanyl	N/A	15 micrograms/hr	Transdermal fentanyl is **approximately 80 times** as potent as morphine (This is based on studies converting from Morphine to fentanyl. Currently, there are no empirical studies converting fentanyl to morphine).	30mg Oral morphine
Meperidine Meperidine is **not** a recommended drug in a palliative care setting and is to be **avoided**. If a patient with chronic pain is on meperidine, convert patient to an equianalgesic dose of one of the other opioids listed in this table.	300mg of oral meperidine	75mg of parenteral meperidine	Oral Morphine is **about 10 times** more potent than oral meperidine and about twice more potent as parenteral meperidine (mg for mg)	30mg Oral morphine
Created by VJ Periyakoil, MD for Stanford eCampus curriculum: http://endoflife.stanford.edu/M11_pain_control/equivalency_table.html				

Vyjeyanthi (VJ) S. Periyakoil, MD, *is a nationally recognized leader in palliative care. She is a clinical associate professor of medicine at Stanford University of Medicine and the director of the Stanford Palliative Care Education & Training Program. She also serves as the Associate Director of Palliative Care Services, VAPAHCS. Her research focuses on health and the health care of adult patients with chronic and serious illnesses, multi-cultural health, geriatrics, ethno-geriatrics, and ethno-palliative care. She is the founder and the director of Stanford eCampus and the director of the Stanford Internet based Successful Aging (http://geriatrics.stanford.edu), a web-based mini fellowship for health personnel from all disciplines as well as lay health advisors, patient navigators, and peer health promoters.*

REFERENCES

Amir, M., Kaplan, Z., Ephron, R., Levine, Y., Benjamin, J., & Kilter, M. (1997). Coping styles in post-traumatic stress disorder (PTSD) patients. *Personality and Individual Difference, 23,* 399–405.

Boscarino, J.A. (2008, July). A prospective study of PTSD and early-age heart disease mortality among Vietnam veterans: Implications for surveillance and prevention. *Psychosomatic Medicine, 70*(6), 668-76.

Breslau, N., Davis, G.C., Andreski, P., & Peterson, E. (1991). Traumatic events and post-traumatic stress disorder in an urban population of young adults. *Archives of General Psychiatry, 48,* 216–222.

Bryant, R.A., & Harvey, A.G. (1995). Avoidant coping style and post-traumatic stress following motor vehicle accidents. *Behaviour Research and Therapy, 33,* 631–635.

Chassen, C., Butler, L., Koopman, C., Miller, E., DiMiceli, S., Giese-Davis, J.,...Spiegel, S. (2001, May). Supportive-Expressive Group Therapy and Distress in Patients With Metastatic Breast Cancer: A Randomized Clinical Intervention Trial. *Archives of General Psychiatry, 58,* 494 – 501

Chilcoat, H.D., & Breslau, N. (1998). Posttraumatic Stress Disorder and Drug Disorders. *Archives of General Psychiatry, 55,* 913-917.

Deykin, E.Y., & Buka, S.L. (1997). Prevalence and risk factors for posttraumatic stress disorder among chemically dependent adolescents. *American Journal of Psychiatry, 154,* 752-757

Jacobsen, L.K., Southwick, S.M., & Kosten, T.R. (2001). Substance use disorders in patients with Posttraumatic Stress Disorder: A review of the literature. *American Journal of Psychiatry, 158*(8), 1184-1190.

Manchikanti, L. (2006, July). *Prescription drug abuse: What is being done to address this drug epidemic?* Statement Before the Sub-Committee on Criminal Justice, Drug Policy, And Human Resources. Washington, DC.

O'Neil, C.K., Hanlon, J.T., & Marcum, Z.A. (2012) Adverse effects of analgesics commonly used by older adults with osteoarthritis: Focus on non-opioid and opioid analgesics. *American Journal of Geriatric Pharmacotherapy, 10*(6), 331-42.

Periyakoil, V.S., Kraemer, H.C., & Noda, A. (2012) Measuring grief and depression in seriously ill outpatients using the Palliative Grief Depression Scale. *Journal of Palliative Medicine, 15*(12), 1350-1355.

Periyakoil, V.S. (2012). Differentiating grief and depression in patients who are seriously ill. *American Family Physician, 86*(3), 232-234.

Saxon, A.J., Davis, T.M., Sloan, K.L., McKnight, K.M., McFall, M.E., & Kivlahan, D.R. (2001). Trauma, symptoms of Posttraumatic Stress Disorder, and associated problems among incarcerated veterans. *Psychiatric Services, 52*(7), 959-964.

Schnurr, P.P., Friedman, M.J., Foy, D.W., Shea, M.T., Hsieh, F.Y., Lavori, PW... Bernardy, N.C. (2003). Randomized trial of trauma-focused group therapy for posttraumatic stress disorder. *Archives of General Psychiatry, 60*, 481-9.

Tan, G., Teo, I., Anderson, K.O., & Jensen, M.P. (2011). Adaptive versus maladaptive coping and beliefs and their relation to chronic pain adjustment. *Clinical Journal of Pain, 27*(9), 769-74.

Taylor, S., Thordarson, D.S., Maxfield, L., Fedoroff, I.C., Lovell, K., & Ogrodniczuk, J. (2003). Comparative efficacy, speed, and adverse effects of three PTSD treatments: Exposure therapy, EMDR, and relaxation training. *Journal of Consulting and Clinical Psychology, 71*(2), 330-8.

Weissman, D.E. (2006, July). *Fast Facts and Concepts #69: Is it pain or addiction?* 2nd Edition. July 2006. Retrieved from End-of-Life / Palliative Education Resource Center: http://www.eperc.mcw.edu/fastFact/ff_69.htm

CHAPTER 12

Voices
The Survivalist. Or Tired and Brave.

Nicky Quinlan

O ur first meeting was formal, brusque, short-sighted even, and perhaps easier on both of us that way. He was welcoming but clear: he had little time for wasters. Mr. H was not ready to consider other paths of living, or dying; this was the survivalist in him.

Mr. H had acute myeloid leukemia. His outlook from this most aggressive disease was tenuous, yet he clung to the rigors of the plan. Obliterative chemotherapy would wipe out all his blood cell lines, and then, if remission was achieved, treatment would proceed to bone marrow transplantation in a distant state (the VA has only three centers that offer this procedure, spread across the United States). The primary medical team had consulted us for symptom management, such as pain and fatigue, but it quickly transpired they needed more support in not only caring *for* him but also caring *about* him. You see, Mr. H was a "challenging patient."

Mr. H introduced me to his IV stand, "Stanley." Truly, it was a tumultuous relationship between them. Stanley would frequently disturb him at night; all it took was a single shrill beep to cut across the stagnant air of his hospital room and shatter his rest. Manacled to his arm, one could sense Stanley's threatening air; a slim sterile pole glinting under a Medusa-like chaos of lines and drips. Yet, Stanley would always be there for him, literally a constant and enduring crutch for those initial weeks after diagnosis. Stanley was there until he was no longer there. And when Stanley left there was grief, but also resolution and freedom.

Napoleon Bonaparte noted "The first virtue in a soldier is endurance of fatigue; courage is only the second virtue." Mr. H had initially presented with prolonged intolerable fatigue, to the point where he could not get out of bed. His son, who had become increasingly alarmed at his father's physical and psychological decline, shouldered his father's broad frame to the local veterans' urgent care. Initial blood tests showed a profound anemia, red cell counts barely compatible with a pulse. The work-up and transition to treatment was swift and efficient; perhaps, in retrospect, too efficient. The enormity of his diagnosis and dire prognosis appeared to get lost in the maelstrom of chemotherapies and their ensuing complications. Time was not for wasting.

As a team we were concerned most with his psychological frailty. Despite attentive medical care, he became increasingly isolated, stranded in his room. When prompted to take a short respite in the corridor or under the hospital's foyer awning for some fresh air he persistently refused, citing his suppressed immune system vulnerable to attack from "critters" unseen. There was some truth in this reasoning but, on balance, we considered it healthier to take this risk. Knowing his son was his father's greatest ally, we worked with him to make a simple plan of exposure therapy. Alas, he declined to move.

Our conversations were like confessionals, intimate by proximity but minus the subtext of sin or guilt. In his darkened room in low tones we would talk; I would mostly listen. I would like to think this was a conspiracy of empathy. Flat on his back his wide shoulders took up much of the bed. Or, bowed and hunched exhaustedly on the edge of bed, he would recount manifold symptoms. His stare was searching, piercing yet paradoxically knowing. Ultimately what he craved most was patience and presence with him through the torment of leukemia, treatment, and uncertainty.

There were echoes from his combat experience, shadows of trauma untold. For decades he had lived a solitary life in the woods of rural New England. Many miles on a dirt track to his cabin, by all accounts he was set up for Armageddon. His adult son from a distant, almost forgotten divorce lived locally; a respected fireman, it was clear they enjoyed each other's company. Visiting with his son was the bright chink in Mr. H's otherwise confined existence. Reloading was their hobby, packing gunpowder in spent bullet casings. Frugal yet dangerous, repetitive but satisfying, it was both science and art. This was one of my salient lessons from Mr. H: simple things we like to do and share with others make all the difference when everything else has been stripped away.

Mr. H was a Vietnam veteran but his past was a tightly sealed chest. He acknowledged a remote history of alcoholism that ended with his ruined marriage. PTSD was a concern. One night in his self-imposed cocoon he experienced a vivid nightmare. A tall female nurse leaned imperiously over him. Wagging her index finger she curtly told him to "settle down, settle down." Perhaps a relic of PTSD from military training or combat experience, the depth of his fear was disturbing. This standoff would intrude especially at times when he felt most vulnerable; when the night before was particularly fragmented or when his back was hurting more. At times he would believe it had really happened, and his insight fluctuated in direct relation to his reserve. Elements of paranoia crept in other times. He believed the antibiotics themselves were the main cause of his insomnia. To test his hypothesis medications were switched twice with little success. What did work effectively, however, was minimizing nighttime disruptions and frontloading his day with the medical activities. A simple intervention, this improved his quality of life immensely in the ensuing weeks.

Mr. H had pain. A robust, lumbering mass of a man, his whole being now ached with fatigue and stiffness. Diffuse central back discomfort was initially difficult to control but improved with scheduled long-acting opiates. Constipation, another iatrogenic burden, compounded his frustration and sense of powerlessness. It became the bogey in his sights; cunning, harassing, but a target never the less. Remarkably, his sense of humor flickered through at the most unexpected moments. His faith in us, however, waxed and waned like a delirium of trust and distrust. Not used to being looked after, he did not adjust well to the role of patient. Frequent and multiple demands became a challenge for many of his caregivers, and burned bridges with some of the staff. Ostensibly he trusted me but had no qualms about showing me the door when he was done. We do not have to like our patients. We do have to treat them equally and without judgment.

Finally, closure. The bone marrow biopsy performed four weeks after induction showed persistent immature white cells. The chemotherapy had failed. If anything, it had made that last month a living hell for him. He had barely survived physically; psychologically he was a battered shell. For a month he had been haunted by pain, insomnia, anxiety, isolation, and the unknown. Now he was free. Free to go home and spend the rest of his days as he wanted. Free from Stanley. Free to sleep without intrusion. A referral was made to home hospice and, with that, he was gone from the room. His prognosis was expected to be short. At our team debriefing, the relief for Mr. H was palpable. He now had some essence of control again. Perhaps he knew some of what was ahead; he was no longer second-guessing.

And through it all, the self-imposed isolation, the needing (as distinct from neediness), and the darkness, Mr. H showed us that, in the face of the most serious illness, while he may not live long, he would survive his way. In that time of unknowing he utilized the skills he had honed in Vietnam and in the remote woods. Survival was not just a matter of life and death.

Editor's Note: The views expressed in this article are those of the author and do not necessarily reflect the position or policy of the Department of Veterans Affairs or the United States government.

Nicky Quinlan *is an Irish doctor, trained in geriatric medicine in Ireland and in Boston, and is currently completing a palliative medicine research fellowship at Stanford University. His research interests are in the geriatric syndrome of frailty, in particular improving frailty recognition and communication with older adults at the end of life.*

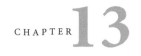

Caring for Seriously Ill Veterans in the Community: Communication, Collaboration, and Coordination

Diane H. Jones

> *We in the VA depend on you, community hospice agencies, to deliver home care for our terminally ill patients. The VA does not intend to replicate the excellent system that is already in place for home hospice care and we in the VA must learn to collaborate with and learn from you.*
> ~Tom Edes, MD, director, Geriatrics and Extended Care Operations, Department of Veterans Affairs

The mission of the Department of Veterans Affairs (VA) Hospice and Palliative Care (HPC) program is to "Honor Veterans' preferences for care at the end of life," whether hospice and palliative services are delivered directly by VA or a community provider. The quote from Dr. Edes demonstrates VA's commitment to collaborate with community providers by promoting smooth transitions across care settings, providing veteran-specific education and training to its community partners, and teaching veterans and their families about the healthcare and benefits they have earned through their service to our country. This chapter will look at the history of VA programs supporting veterans at the end of life, as well as current programs and models both within VA and other healthcare organizations.

These programs facilitate communication, collaboration, and coordination of care and benefits for veterans across VA and community settings. The approach is veteran-centric in that it focuses on the needs, desires, and treatment of our veterans and their families. This chapter provides information about VA and community collaborations, the unique needs veterans may have as they approach the end of their lives, the complex interface between VA and the community, and ways in which Hospice-Veteran Partnerships can help overcome these challenges in pursuit of honoring veterans' preferences.

BACKGROUND

Every hospice in this country has cared for veterans at some time, whether or not they know it. In 2012 about 642,000 veteran deaths are predicted nationally, representing greater than one quarter of all deaths in the United States (www.va.gov/vetdata). In 2011, a little over 3% or approximately 21,000 veterans died in VA facilities. This means that the vast majority of veterans dying in the community are receiving care from providers that may be unaware of their military history and the special needs related to their experience. In addition, most veterans are not enrolled in the VA healthcare system, and many may not be aware of their VA, Medicare, or other third-party payer hospice benefits. Community providers can facilitate connections that help eligible veterans enroll in VA and access the services they have earned, including survivors' benefits for eligible family members.

Currently the largest age group of veteran deaths is 80 to 89 years old, having served during World War II and the Korean Conflict. Demographics are rapidly changing; by 2014, 60% of veterans over the age of 65 and 22% of all veteran deaths will be Vietnam-era veterans. As Deborah Grassman, author of *Peace at Last: Stories of Hope and Healing for Veterans and Their Families*, (2009) writes, there is much we need to learn in order to meet the needs of this special population, including how Posttraumatic Stress Disorder (PTSD) and substance abuse affect care at the end of life. For all veterans in general and particularly those involved in the Vietnam era, hospice staff may be the healthcare providers who have the last opportunity, and the privilege, to help provide closure and simply say, "Thank you for your service to our country."

CREATING A VETERAN-CENTRIC CULTURE

Military culture and training influences a soldier's life and death. War may leave men and women with physical and mental wounds. Posttraumatic stress symptoms may also surface at the end of life, requiring specific clinical competencies to address veteran-specific physical, emotional, spiritual, and psychosocial symptoms. On the other hand, military experiences and relationships may be a source of strength and comfort. These two realities of how military culture may impact the end of life make it essential to build and maintain relationships across VA and community settings, create Vet-to-Vet volunteer programs, and involve Veteran Service Organizations.

Knowing which of your patients are veterans is the first step to creating a veteran-centric culture. Knowing what to do with the information is key to creating a culture within your organization that has the capacity and competency to honor veterans' preferences while meeting their physical, social, emotional, and spiritual needs. This requires active participation, communication, coordination and collaboration with VA and other community healthcare providers.

Focuses on the needs, desires, and treatment of our veterans

VA's Uniform Benefits Package includes access to hospice and palliative care for all enrolled veterans (38 CFR 17.36 and 17.38). Community hospices can honor veterans' preferences by knowing their veteran patients' goals of care, including the setting of their choice. This is often at home but can include returning to a VA facility for inpatient care. A dually-eligible veteran enrolled in both the Veterans Health Administration (VHA) and Medicare has the right to access both systems simultaneously, creating "open access" to hospice and palliative care (VHA Handbook 1140.5). In order to serve veterans, community providers need to know the rules and regulations as well as how to help veterans access services to which they are entitled.

Requires veteran responsibility and accountability

In order for veterans to make decisions about their own end-of-life care, they must first be aware of services and benefits they are eligible to receive. Community providers can plan and participate in outreach activities such as talking to veterans' groups, developing brochures that focus on hospice benefits for veterans, taking part in "Stand Downs" (collaborative one-to-three day events providing services to homeless veterans coordinated between local VAs, other government agencies, and community agencies), and educating other community providers about the needs veterans may have at the end of life. Community hospice providers are especially trained to help patients identify their goals of care but must be knowledgeable about veterans' issues to engage successfully with this population.

Depends on communication, coordination, and collaboration among healthcare providers

VA is committed to partnering with community providers and has made it a top priority (*Strategic Plan Refresh FY 2011-2015*, Department of Veterans Affairs), encouraging community providers and VA staff to establish relationships and together develop processes to ensure smooth transitions across settings and venues of care. By staying focused on what the veteran needs, VA and community providers can hold joint educational events, identify and solve local challenges, and create processes focused on veterans and their needs.

COMMUNICATION

To effectively serve veterans, community and government organizations must identify each other, develop strong lines of communication across all venues of care and services, and establish internal and external programs to reach out to veterans. Hospice-Veteran Partnerships (HVP) offer a good place for VA and community providers to start working together to learn about each other and reach out to veterans. Other activities can also help develop relationships with veterans and their families; more information can be found later in this chapter.

Veterans talk to other veterans. When thinking about reaching out to them, first identify veterans in your own organization who may be able to provide insight and perspective. If you use volunteers, recruit and train veterans in the community to create your own volunteer Vet-to-Vet program. These volunteers can assist veteran patients/clients as well as speak to Veterans' Service Organizations like the Veterans of Foreign Wars and other government and non-government organizations serving veterans.

Veterans Health Administration (VHA) Organization

Organizationally, the first step in establishing good lines of communication with VA staff is developing a working knowledge of the basic structure of the Veterans Health Administration (VHA), a broad understanding of the services it provides and how it interfaces with Medicare and the community. VHA is one of three administrations in VA – the other two are the Veterans Benefits Administration (VBA) and the National Cemetery Administration (NCA) – and is the largest integrated healthcare system in the country. It is a complex system with many layers of authority, levels of service, and rules and regulations. It is perceived by many providers and consumers to be an "impenetrable fortress", inaccessible to the community and sometimes even to veterans.

VHA is divided into 21 regions or Veterans Integrated Service Networks (VISNs) to align resources and meet veterans' health care needs. Although VISNs are organized geographically, some VISNs cover more than one state, and some states are covered by more than one VISN (see Figure 1).

Because VISN boundaries do not correspond to state boundaries, establishing effective channels of communication is complex and sometimes cumbersome. Community hospices may not know which VA facility to contact or who in the facility can best help with the various issues that may arise in coordinating care between VA and the private sector. For example, West Virginia has four VISNs (VISNs 4, 5, 6, and 9) and VISN 1 includes six states (ME, NH, VT, MA, RI, CT).

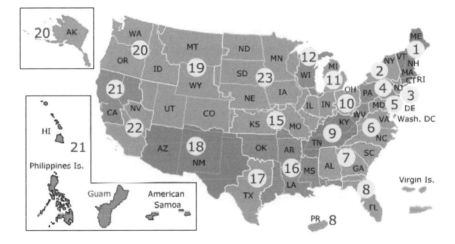

Figure 1. Map of the Veterans Health Administration
(http://www2.va.gov/directory/guide/division_flsh.asp?dnum=1)

VA Medical Centers (VAMCs) are hospital systems that serve veterans. Although the exact makeup of these systems will vary, many have more than one campus and most include ambulatory care and outpatient clinics, nursing home care programs, home care programs, and long-term care domiciliaries. VA medical centers are organized under VISNs.

VA Community-Based Outpatient Clinics (CBOCs) provide outpatient medical care to veterans and are organized under VA medical centers. Most do not have a palliative care program in place; referrals to community hospices for VA-paid hospice care often must go through a designated staff person at the VAMC of jurisdiction.

Vet Centers serve veterans and their families by providing a continuum of quality care that adds value for veterans, families, and communities. Care includes professional readjustment counseling, bereavement counseling, community education, outreach to special populations, brokering services with community agencies, and providing a key access link between veterans and other services in VA.

The VHA Palliative Care Consult Team (PCCT) Directive, first released in 2003 and reissued in 2008, requires every VA facility to ensure that a fully functioning PCCT is implemented as part of each facility's Palliative Care Program (VHA Directives 2003-008 and 2008-066). PCCTs may provide direct and consulting services throughout the VA hospital and in outpatient settings such as a cardiology, oncology, or pain clinic. A growing number of VA facilities are establishing outpatient Palliative Care Clinics, which are often managed by the PCCT or in conjunction with one of the other clinics. These clinics help veterans manage their pain and other symptoms and coordinate their care with both inpatient and other outpatient services like Home-Based Primary Care. Some VA Outpatient Palliative Care clinics are located adjacent to or are part of a VA hospital site, while others may be freestanding and located many miles from the VA hospital. Remotely located outpatient clinics are affiliated with a parent VA hospital. Facility PCCT coordinators are often the point of contact for community providers.

Medicare Hospice Benefit and veterans' hospice benefits

Good, effective communication also includes having a grasp of the relationship between the Medicare Hospice Benefit and VA-paid hospice services. Veterans enrolled in both Medicare and VHA are dually eligible for both VA benefits and Medicare benefits. By policy, they can choose to have either Medicare or VA pay for hospice services. If they choose Medicare to pay for hospice, they still retain all of their health care benefits from VA.

Veterans who are not enrolled in Medicare but are enrolled in VA can access all of their VA benefits, including VA-paid hospice. Sometimes an admitting hospice will identify a veteran who is not enrolled in VA, in which case they can initiate an expedited enrollment process through the Catastrophic Coverage directive (VHA Directive 2009-073). Hospice staff should contact the palliative care coordinator at their veteran's VA facility for help. Once enrolled in VA, the veteran must be referred to VA-paid hospice by a VA physician.

COLLABORATION

Understanding VA

Successful relationships are based on appreciating the organizational cultures, roles, funding sources, governance, and accountability that each party brings to the table. What follows is a brief discussion of VA's culture that can provide some insight into a very complex organization and help community hospices engage in respectful, productive collaborations.

Culture: VA staff work in a quasi-military environment where there is an expectation that orders will be followed throughout the chain of command. VA staff care for those who served in the military, so there is a strong sense of respect, honor, and duty. VA staff, like most healthcare providers, are very protective of their patients and concerned that outside organizations may not know how to give veterans the care they need. Developing expertise in meeting the unique needs of seriously ill veterans goes a long way in cementing a good working relationship with VA staff.

Role: VA is first and foremost a provider of acute, long-term and outpatient care in a variety of settings. When a veteran chooses VA-paid hospice care, VA becomes a payer as well, which requires that the VA facility refer the veteran to a Medicare-certified hospice that is an approved vendor. Referrals for veterans electing the Medicare Hospice Benefit do not require a formal agreement and can be made to the hospice of the veteran's choice or on a rotating basis using a list of community providers.

The distinction between provider and payer is an important concept for community hospices to understand when they are working with VA facilities. As a provider, VA physicians and other clinical staff appreciate regular updates on the status of their patients and notification when the veteran has died. As a payer, designated VA staff need to approve admissions, changes in levels of care, and inpatient hospital stays.

There are sharp lines of demarcation between VA staff who provide clinical care, those who refer to community agencies, those who negotiate vendor agreements, and those who pay the bills. As in many hospitals, these staff may not know each other, may not have any regular contact, and may work on separate campuses miles away. The best approach for community hospices interested in fostering a relationship with a local VA facility is to learn the VA system and jargon, find out who is responsible for what, and engage in discussions with the appropriate person(s).

Funding: VA's budget is appropriated by Congress and funds are allocated to VA facilities from their respective VISN of jurisdiction. The budget is fixed and priorities are often set by Congress. VA facilities vary considerably in how they choose to spend their budgeted funds, depending on local values, needs, and availability of resources.

Accountability: VA reports regularly to Congress and is ultimately accountable to the President of the United States. It is required to respond quickly to demands for data and other information. The VA Office of Inspector General is responsible for oversight of VA. Federal employees are not permitted to lobby elected officials, solicit funds, or do anything that might be construed as attempts to influence policy makers.

We Honor Veterans

We Honor Veterans (*WHV*) is a national hospice provider awareness campaign conducted by the National Hospice and Palliative Care Organization (NHPCO) in collaboration with VA's Hospice and Palliative Care program. The campaign focuses on respectful inquiry, compassionate listening, and grateful acknowledgment to better serve our nation's veterans at the end of life. Since its inception, almost 2,000 hospices across the United States have enrolled as WHV Partners.

WHV provides educational tools and resources for hospices, state hospice organizations, Hospice-Veteran Partnerships and VA facilities to:
- Promote veteran-centric educational activities,
- Increase organizational capacity to serve veterans,
- Support development of strategic partnerships, and
- Increase access and improve quality of care.

Hospice-Veteran Partnerships

Hospice-Veteran Partnerships (HVPs) are a key component in the *We Honor Veterans* campaign. Organized as coalitions of people and organizations, stakeholders come together to facilitate veterans' access to high-quality end-of-life care in the community and promote seamless transition among VA facilities, State Veterans Homes, and the community. HVPs can play a significant part now and into the future by increasing the clinical competency of VA and community providers, engaging in educational and outreach efforts for all veterans, and elevating the general public's awareness of veterans in our society.

Successful HVPs are often state-based and "housed" in the state hospice organization, a statewide end-of-life coalition, or a VA medical center; leadership is provided by representatives from community hospices and VA facilities. Statewide HVPs often encourage and support the formation of "local HVPs" that generally are organized within a VA facility's catchment area. Indeed, many statewide HVPs have been started through the local efforts of existing relationships between a VA facility and one or more community hospices.

When forming an HVP and considering potential partners, it is important to think about any and all groups that have contact with veterans. The core group includes VA facilities, community hospices and end-of-life coalitions in the state, State Veterans Homes, Veterans Service Organizations, and community veterans' organizations. Remember, each HVP is unique, so both emerging and established HVPs should strive to include whatever partners can best reach veterans in their area.

Successful HVPs generally have strong support from VA, both at the facility and VISN levels. They have at least one champion from each facility in the state at their HVP table. They have invited staff from CBOCs, State Veterans Homes, and perhaps Vet Centers, to participate. They have found that there is strength in numbers, and having facility and community-based VA staff involved gives everyone an opportunity to learn from each other. This level of communication also helps to create a common understanding of VA hospice services and referral processes.

Statewide and local HVPs are successful at addressing and solving issues such as: lack of shared knowledge about the different systems of benefits and healthcare available to veterans; misunderstandings about referral processes among healthcare providers and payment for hospice services; and difficulties in caring for veterans across settings of care. Through local, state and regional education events and targeted outreach activities, members of HVPs are learning that together they can improve access, continuity, and quality of end-of-life care for all veterans (Jones, Edes, and Casarett, 2006).

State Veterans Homes

State Veterans Homes (SVH) are the largest deliverer of long-term care to our nation's veterans, and all combined, have more nursing home beds than VHA. They provide care for veterans disabled by age, disease, or disability and incapable of earning a living. Community hospices have had varying degrees of success in collaborating with SVHs, partly because of misunderstandings of the rules and regulations guiding each entity.

It is important to understand that SVHs are not part of VA's healthcare system. Representing federal-state partnerships, they are owned and operated by the state and are regulated by federal and state laws. Because they receive per diem payments from VA for enrolled veterans and grants for capital expenditures, federal law requires annual inspection by the VA Medical Center of jurisdiction. Some states contract out management responsibilities to a private management company and SVH staff may or may not be employees of the company. Other states may operate their SVHs through the state's Department of Military and Veterans Affairs, Department of Health, or other departments. To get more information about each state's programs, visit www.va.gov/statedva.htm.

Unlike VA, there is no national headquarters from which SVHs' policies, standards, and compliance are centralized and promoted. Instead, each state is responsible for its own veterans nursing homes with VA providing federally-prescribed support through the grant programs and oversight through annual inspections.

Eligibility is established through both federal and state laws. The federal law covers veterans, their spouses, and Gold Star parents who have lost a child during military service as defined in Title 38 United States Code, Section 101. Under this Code, the term "veteran" means a person who served in the active military, naval, or air service, and who was discharged or released under conditions other than dishonorable.

Veterans Service Officers

More and more community hospices are discovering the importance of collaborating with Veterans Service Organizations and County Veteran Service Officers, both of whom are advocates for veterans and their dependents.

- Veterans Service Organizations include Veterans of Foreign Wars, American Legion, and many others. For a list of all of the VSOs and their national offices, visit www.va.gov/vso. Note: Most VSOs have state and/or local chapters with members ready to help their fellow veterans.

- State and County Veterans Service Officers generally have similar responsibilities, but may be paid by the state and county, respectively. County Veterans Service Officers are local government employees that are county or town based and can be a great asset to community providers seeking to assist veterans and their families in accessing benefits.

COORDINATION

Working with VA

Many of our veterans may not be aware of the services to which they are entitled. Providers of care and services for veterans may not be knowledgeable about the unique needs of veterans at the end of life or how to help them and their families access the care they need. Eligibility for hospice in VA is very similar to the eligibility requirements for the Medicare Hospice Benefit. In addition to diagnosis and prognosis requirements veterans must be enrolled in VA in order to access hospice in VA Medical Centers as well as VA-paid hospice services in the community.

In order to be reimbursed for care, community hospice providers must be Medicare-certified and an approved vendor by the VA facility authorizing the services. The process for becoming an approved vendor is determined by individual VA facilities. Hospices must also confirm a veteran's enrollment status in VA and secure authorization from the veteran's physician prior to starting services. If the veteran is not enrolled in VA, community hospice providers can contact the nearest VA facility PCCT coordinator or Eligibility Department to explore the possibility of an expedited enrollment.

Definition of "Veteran"

One of the most basic issues to address is seemingly simple: the definition of "veteran." But asking the question, "Are you a veteran?" has the potential to be confusing to both veterans and their families, because not all people that have served in the military consider themselves to be a veteran. They may believe, for example, that they must have served during a time of war or conflict, or served outside of the United States in order to call themselves a veteran. The better choice may be to ask, "Did you serve in the military?" This will help them answer the question in a way that staff can complete an assessment and assist in identifying benefits for which veterans and family members may be eligible.

The Federal Benefits for Veterans, Dependents and Survivors booklet states, "Eligibility for most VA benefits is based upon discharge from active military service under other than dishonorable conditions" (2012, p. 12). Dishonorable and bad-conduct discharges issued by general courts-martial may bar VA benefits. Veterans in prison and parolees must contact a VA regional office to determine eligibility. VA benefits will not be provided to any veteran or dependent wanted for an outstanding felony warrant.

Community hospices and other community providers should explore the individual's perceptions of his or her service to our country. For the purposes of providing care, the fact that there is a history of having served in the U.S. Armed Forces or National Guard is very relevant and not necessarily related to discharge status except if the provider is seeking veteran's benefits for the patient. Any military history, including a less than honorable discharge, may produce lingering and difficult emotions that could surface while under the care of the community provider and would need careful attention and skilled intervention.

Understanding and implementing the Military History Checklist

The Military History Checklist is designed to help community hospices identify their veteran patients, evaluate the impact of the military experience, and determine if there are benefits to which the veteran and surviving dependents may be entitled. This section provides information about interpreting and implementing the Military History Checklist, which can be found in the Resource section of this book.

Community providers can integrate all or parts of the Military History Checklist into the interdisciplinary team intake process, tailoring the questions to fit their culture and patient needs. Hospices are beginning to work with vendors to include the questions in their hospice software programs, allowing them to track their veteran patients separately. Learning to use the Military History Checklist takes time and training. A good place to start is to review the Military History Checklist Guide, optimally with someone with military experience or VA staff.

Veteran-specific education

VA's Hospice and Palliative Care program partnered with Education in Palliative and End-of-Life Care (EPEC), End-of-Life Nursing Education Consortium (ELNEC), and the Hospice and Palliative Nurses Association (HPNA), to develop veteran-specific curricula for use in VA and to share with the community. All of these curricula are in the public domain and are available online through the websites found at the Resource section at the end of this book.

The EPEC for Veterans Project adapted the EPEC Curriculum, creating a 22-module veteran-specific curriculum complete with trigger tapes. Similar to EPEC, the ELNEC-For-Veterans curriculum was adopted from their core ELNEC curriculum. The Hospice Education Network (HEN) has partnered with ELNEC to provide the ELNEC - For Veterans curriculum online.

HPNA developed two Palliative Care Nursing Assistants (PCNA) curricula to prepare registered nurses to teach nursing assistants and to provide web-based veteran-specific modules that can be accessed by nursing assistants and other staff. These free programs include topics such as *Communicating with Veterans at the End of Life, Pain Management at the End of Life for Veterans,* and *Care of the Veteran: Spiritual Distress.*

Quality improvement

The Family Evaluation of Hospice Care-Veterans (FEHC-V) survey is a version of the Family Evaluation of Hospice Care (FEHC) survey that includes questions related to care targeted specifically to veterans and their family caregivers. These veteran-specific questions are grouped in a separate section (Section V) and have been placed at the end of the regular FEHC survey questions.

The VA Bereaved Family Survey (BFS), like FEHC-V, measures aspects of bereaved family satisfaction with end-of-life care for enrolled veterans. However, the BFS is administered to family members of veterans who died as inpatients in VA facilities. Items in the BFS cover areas of care such as communication, emotional and spiritual support, pain management and personal care needs. Additional open-ended items are included in the BFS to give family members the opportunity to provide comments regarding the care the patient received. The BFS survey results provide valuable input on the quality of care delivered by VA as well as opportunities for grieving family members to access bereavement support and benefits. Additional information about the survey and its methods can be found at: www.cherp.research.va.gov/PROMISE.asp.

Armed with their survey results, members of Hospice-Veteran Partnerships or VA facility staff and their hospice vendors can compare the responses to the survey questions across settings and identify areas in which they are doing well, as well as areas that would benefit from quality improvement actions. Below is a comparison of FEHC-V and BFS questions that can be compared across VA and community settings.

A comparison of FEHC-V and BFS questions

NHPCO FEHC-V Questions	CA Bereaved Family Survey Questions
#2 How often did the hospice staff take the time to listen to the patient's stories and/or concerns related to his/her military experiences?	#1 During [Veteran's] last month, how much of the time were the doctors and other staff who took care of [Veteran] willing to take time to listen? (Always)
#3 Some Veterans near the end of life re-experience the stress and emotions that they had when they were in combat. Did this happen to the patient? (if no, skip to # 6)	#9 Some Veterans near the end of life re-experience the stress and emotions that they had when they were in combat. Did this happen to the [Veteran] in the last month of life? (% Yes)
#4 How often did the patient's combat related stress make him/her uncomfortable?	#10 How often did [Veteran's] stress make him/ her uncomfortable in the last month of life? {PTSD} (% Never)
#6 Would it have been helpful to have more information about VA benefits for surviving spouses and dependents?	#14 Would it have been helpful if the VA had provided more information about benefits for surviving spouses and dependents? (% No)
#7 Would it have been helpful to have more information about VA burial and memorial benefits?	#15 Would it have been helpful if the VA had provided more information about burial and memorial benefits? (% No)

SUMMARY

Veteran-centric practices can be integrated into a hospice agency's culture through communication, collaboration, and coordination. A number of programs exist that have developed tools and resources, in order to help organizations at the community level open gateways to promote active, productive, and effective partnering.

Editor's Note: The views expressed in this chapter do not necessarily express the views of the Department of Veterans Affairs or the United States Government.

Diane H. Jones, *MSW, is the co-founder and president of Ethos Consulting Group, L.L.C. Ms. Jones has had more than 30 years of experience in the field of hospice and palliative care, and for more than 14 years she has consulted with the Department of Veterans Affairs (VA) providing administrative and management assistance with national projects related to improving access to end-of-life care for our nation's veterans. She would like to thank NHPCO, its Veterans Advisory Council, and the countless VA and community hospice providers that worked with them, for creating the* Hospice-Veteran Partnership Toolkit, *the* VA 101 Toolkit, *and the* Military History Toolkit, *all of which greatly contributed to the content of this chapter.*

REFERENCES

Department of Veterans Affairs. *Strategic plan refresh FY 2011-2015.* Retrieved from http://www.va.gov/

Department of Veteran Affairs. (2012). *The federal benefits for Veterans, dependents and survivors.* Retrieved from http://www.va.gov/opa/publications/benefits_book/benefits_introduction.asp

Grassman, D.L. (2009). *Peace at last: Stories of hope and healing for veterans and their families.* St. Petersburg, FL: Vandamere Press.

Jones, D., Edes, T., & Casarett, D. (2006). You won't know if you're improving unless you measure: Recommendations for evaluating Hospice-Veteran Partnerships. *Journal of Pain and Symptom Management, 32*(5), 488-496.

CHAPTER 14

Programs that Work: *We Honor Veterans*

I t surprises many Americans to learn that 25% of all deaths in the United States are veterans. That's 1,800 people a day, more than 680,000 veterans every year. These heroic Americans deserve recognition for their military service, particularly at the end of life's journey.

All hospices are serving veterans but often aren't aware that many of those they are caring for have served in the armed forces. By recognizing the unique needs of our nation's veterans who are facing a life-limiting illness, professional caregivers are able to accompany and guide veterans and their families toward a more peaceful ending.

In September 2010, the National Hospice and Palliative Care Organization, in collaboration with the Department of Veterans Affairs (VA), launched *We Honor Veterans (WHV)*, a pioneering program to help improve the care veterans receive from hospice and palliative care providers.

The program's centerpiece is the *We Honor Veterans* website, where staff can learn more about the special needs of veterans, find tools and resources to assist with education, and become a *WHV* Partner.

The website, www.WeHonorVeterans.org, provides staff, state hospice organizations, and Hospice-Veteran Partnerships with tools and resources that encourage them to:

- Learn more about caring for veterans;
- Declare a commitment to honoring veterans at the end of life;
- Partner with VA at the local, regional and national level; and
- Measure quality and outcomes for continued improvement.

There are four Partner Levels, based on demonstrated work and progressive commitment to serving veterans. Each Partner Level guides the staff through education and activities that progressively increase their ability to serve veterans. The four levels and their primary goals:

Level 1 Partner: Provide veteran-centric education for staff and volunteers, and identify patients with military experience.

Level 2 Partner: Build organizational capacity to provide quality care for veterans.

Level 3 Partner: Develop and strengthen relationships with VA medical centers and other veteran organizations.

Level 4 Partner: Increase access and improve quality of care for veterans.

As each Partner Level is achieved, the organization is awarded a distinctive Partner logo which can be used to symbolize—and celebrate—enhanced end-of-life care and services to veterans.

There are almost 2,000 hospices which participate in the program and are recognizing veterans in a variety of creative and, often heartfelt, ways. What impact is it making on the care provided to veterans and their families? Below, several *WHV* Partners discuss the initiative they're most proud of and how it is succeeding in recognizing veterans for their service while also improving their quality of life at life's end.

A Small Gesture That Opens Doors
Pikes Peak Hospice & Palliative Care
Colorado Springs, CO

Several years ago, staff members who are veterans themselves, or had served in the uniformed services, initiated a special effort to formally thank the distinguished veterans receiving care. Each veteran patient is presented with an heirloom-quality coin, created in the shape of a "dog tag," and a certificate of appreciation that bears the seal of his or her branch of service. These coins are patterned after the "coins for excellence" that nearly all service members have received while in uniform. While just a piece of metal, the coins of excellence are treasured by all soldiers, sailors, Marines, or airmen who had one pressed into their hands as a "thank you" for service rendered, so it was fitting to model our small gift after them.

This simple act of gratitude opens the door to these veterans' untold stories. Our hospice care teams report again and again that when the coin and certificate are presented, a pent-up dam of emotion bursts. It is profoundly moving to look into the eyes of a veteran whose buddies didn't come back or who has seen what the weapons of modern technology can do to a human body, and see the light begin to shine again.

Creating a Lasting Tribute
Hospice & Palliative CareCenter
Winston-Salem, NC

Last fall, the staff, volunteers, and patients and families of Hospice & Palliative CareCenter were joined by invited guests to unveil their Veterans Garden. The garden is situated in front of the CareCenter's Hospice House on the 14-acre wooded campus. Its centerpiece is a flagpole that is embedded in a large boulder, upon which the emblems of the five branches of military service are engraved. The flagpole is surrounded by a raised flower bed and four custom benches, designed and handcrafted by local sculptors and artists. The benches feature beautiful mosaic designs, some made from actual bullet casings. The garden is designed for wheelchair accessibility, with the goal of being a special place for reflection and respite while also being a tangible expression of thanks to all veterans who have served our country.

Of special note was the overwhelming support received from the community to build the Garden. The fundraising efforts were swift and successful, illustrating the community's shared passion for this project.

As we look upon the finished garden, we see the benefits that have come from it:

- a demonstration of our organizational support of veterans
- a opportunity for members of the community to express their gratitude to service members
- a bridge to establishing and maintaining valuable relationships with the VA, the local chapter of the Veterans of Foreign Wars (VFW), Patriot Guard Riders, and the Oak Ridge Military Academy.

Public Recognition through Community Pinnings
Mercy Care
Myrtle Beach, SC

"We Love Our Vets" read the sign at the Inlet Square Mall in Myrtle Beach. It was Valentine's Day 2012, and Mercy Care had been asked to collaborate on a special event to honor and thank the veterans in our community for their service to the country. Our ambition was to make this the largest pinning to take place in our county.

When Valentine's Day arrived, so did our country's finest. Flags representing all branches of service were carried into the Mall's central court where over 300 hundred family members and guests were seated and watched with pride as their loved ones entered and took their seats. There were bands playing, patriotic songs, and appearances by the JROTC drill team, Rolling Thunder, and the Patriot Guard.

After short speeches to express the community's gratitude for their service, highlighted by a poem written and read by a veteran of the Korean War, the veterans from each branch were asked to stand. Mercy Care veteran volunteers walked through each aisle and carefully placed a specially designed "Mercy HONORS" pin on the lapel of each veteran standing at attention. After veterans from each branch received their pins, the Mercy veteran volunteers stood at attention and saluted each group. One veteran after another smiled with appreciation while others had tears streaming down their cheeks. For many, this was the first time anyone had thanked them for their service. During this event, over 350 veterans were recognized, from World War II through present conflicts in Afghanistan and Iraq.

Great care must be taken to recognize our living veterans, but greater care must be provided to recognize families that have lost a loved one in times of armed conflict. Make it a practice to invite these family members or close friends to stand and be recognized for their sacrifice and loss. To those who stand, say "I am sorry for your loss and I thank you for your family's sacrifice to help protect our freedoms." It is then that healing begins.

The Gift of Veteran Volunteers
Covenant Hospice
Pensacola, FL

Early last summer, two gentlemen had a special conversation about an important last wish. "All I want to do is go to the Naval Aviation Museum. Then I'll never have to leave my home again," Randy told Jim. Randy is an Army veteran and Covenant Hospice patient and Jim is a Navy veteran and Covenant Hospice volunteer. Voicing that wish was all that was needed.

Within a month of that conversation, Randy was at the renowned museum and received a special two-hour tour from Vice Admiral Gerald Hoewing. He was also given a medallion commemorating the 2012 opening of the National Flight Academy and a book detailing the history of the museum. As Randy's handwritten note later expressed, the tour was an experience he will cherish forever. Jim was the catalyst that made it happen.

Veterans have made many sacrifices that undeniably leave a lasting impact on their lives years after they have taken off the uniform. While staff are taught the special needs of veterans through trainings and our close work with the VA and local Veteran Service Organizations, veteran volunteers can be the best teachers, and can make an invaluable contribution in the care provided to our nation's finest at the end of life.

Advocating for the Veteran and Family
VITAS Innovative Hospice Care of Atlanta Metro
Atlanta, GA

In Atlanta's metropolitan area, Larry Robert, the veterans' liaison for VITAS, works closely with VA, Medicare, Medicaid, and local organizations to help ensure that veterans and their families receive the care and benefits to which they are entitled. When admitting veteran patients to the hospice program, Robert, who served 13 years as a Navy chaplain, conducts a special assessment to determine the specific level of support they may need.

Robert, one of Georgia's 15 accredited claims agents with the VA, files claims for veterans directly. "Many veterans aren't aware that they're eligible for benefits from VA, and we work hard to ensure they receive the specialized care they need," he said.

As part of this commitment, Robert and his colleagues at VITAS work closely with other veterans' organizations that VITAS supports. This includes:

- Sponsoring *Keep the Spirit of '45 Alive*, the Tuskegee Airmen, and Honor Flight, which all work to celebrate and honor veterans.
- Working with state and local veterans' groups and organizations to advocate for veterans and ensure they receive the support they need at the end of life.
- Participating in the *Veterans History Project*, which seeks to record and document a living legacy of veterans' stories that are archived at the Library of Congress as living legacy.

These specialized programs and others are critically important for veterans, Robert said. "As they near the end of life, many become almost obsessed with their military history, regardless of whether they spent one year or 60 in the military." For this reason, in addition to providing medical care and emotional support, Robert and the Veterans Program team also provide something very important that veterans need: recognition. "It may be difficult for those who are not veterans to understand this because it might not seem like much, but veterans really need to make peace with their military experience," Robert said. "They just want someone to recognize their service and sacrifices."

*Contributors include **Anne Koepsell**, RN, BSN, MHA, CLNC, Executive Director of Washington State Hospice and Palliative Care Organization, and the **We Honor Veterans staff** of NHPCO. The "Making a Difference" stories are excerpts from the original article "WHV Partners Give Thanks" in the November 2012 issue of NHPCO's NewsLine. Visit www.WeHonorVeterans.org for more information, tools, and resources.*

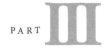

Grief and Loss

O ne of the great insights of the hospice movement was that life-limiting illness was inevitably a family crisis that transcended the individual patient. Thus the family, rather than an individual patient, was the unit of care; care that extends beyond the death to assist the family as they cope with the grief that follows that loss.

Doka's chapter considers the role of ritual and memorials in grief. Doka recounts the rich traditions that surround military funerals as well as the history of memorials. While rituals are generally therapeutic, he describes ways to enhance the value of such rituals such as personalizing the funeral, allowing participation, addressing cultural differences, and acknowledging the multiple identities that frame most lives. In validating the importance of sacred space and sacred ceremonies, Doka notes that the therapeutic value of rituals need not be limited to funerals. Rituals can become part of the therapeutic process used to reaffirm a continuing bond, mark a point of transition in the journey with grief, affirm the significance of the decreased, or to finish unfinished business. Doka also offers a brief sidebar that explores an unfortunate aspect of contemporary military funerals – the possibility of picketing by members of the fringe Westboro Baptist Church.

McGuire's chapter focuses on offering bereavement services to military families. McGuire describes the many factors that can complicate bereavement care, and notes that the shared stoicism of military culture may inhibit seeking bereavement services. McGuire explores how the multiple moves that military families make may limit opportunities for support, particularly for foreign-born spouses. McGuire is especially sensitive how the separations and strains of military life, including the possibility of multiple divorces and families, as well as the stress of combat and possible Posttraumatic Stress Disorder (PTSD), can create difficulties in family relations that can complicate grief.

While the focus of the book is on end-of-life care for veterans, we could not ignore two other types of death that occur in the military–combat deaths and suicide. Harrington-LaMorie and Beard, in their discussion of combat deaths, begin with a central demographic fact; most of the deaths in the military are younger individuals, often between the ages of 18 to 30, who die under violent and traumatic circumstances. Harrington-LaMorie and Beard's chapter is extensive as they describe the numerous factors, such as the condition of the body, that might complicate grief, or the bereavement overload that might result from rapid relocation following a loss. Harrington-LaMorie and Beard are especially sensitive to the nature of death notification, acknowledging that how the reality of death is communicated can be a factor that affects subsequent grief. They also emphasize that grief over a soldier's death may be disenfranchised by others, given the fact that the soldier choose "dangerous work" and thus suffered the consequences. Certainly we also need to remember that another disenfranchised group of grievers are soldiers who served alongside the deceased. As noted throughout the book, camaraderie is one of the more positive aspects of military culture. Yet in the currency of the mission and the throes of combat, the real grief that comrades feel is oft ignored. Harrington-LaMorie and Beard conclude their chapter with implications and resources for grief counseling.

Steen's *Voices* piece powerfully reaffirms the plight that Harrington-LaMorie and Beard describe. Steen not only addresses the traumatic nature of her husband's sudden death but the secondary losses she experienced as well. There is a great gap between a military wife and a military widow. Yet, her story also reaffirms another aspect of Harrington-LaMorie and Beard's chapter; within military culture, there is also resilience.

Leenaars' chapter ends this section. He addresses military suicide, a topic that is garnering more attention each day. Leenaars explores possible reasons for what appears to be an increase in military suicides, as well as discussing programs for prevention, intervention, and postvention.

The section reiterates a central theme; the death of a member or veteran of the armed services affects many. The lesson of hospice care should not be lost; care needs to continue after death.

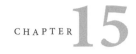

CHAPTER 15

Sacred Ceremonies, Sacred Space: The Role of Rituals and Memorials in Grief and Loss

Kenneth J. Doka

Long before humans could write, our nomadic ancestors would return year after year to the same places to bury and mourn their dead. The ritualistic ways that the dead were buried and the careful place of treasured objects bear mute testimony both to sacredness of the space as well as the ceremony. Their motives have been questioned. Were they honoring their dead? Did they believe that by such careful ritual they would assure their kinsmen and kinswomen successfully journeyed to the other side? Were such rituals meant to placate the dead, to discourage them from returning to trouble the living?

In the end, it does not really matter. Before written history, humans understood the need for memorials and cemeteries–for sacred space and sacred ceremonies.

This lesson too was understood by the military from time immortal. While Plutarch's comment that Spartan mothers told their sons to either return with their shield or on it suggests early rituals, most contemporary rituals that surround military deaths have their origins in the nineteenth century. For example, draping the American flag over the casket of a deceased veteran began with the custom of carrying the dead from the battlefield on flags or draping flags over the bodies of the deceased. The American custom of playing *Taps* at military funerals began during the Civil War. The 21-gun salute was the result of an agreement between the United States and Britain in 1875 to standardize what had been a more idiosyncratic process; the US would often fire a volley for each of the then 21 states in the country. Some military funeral rituals reach even further back into antiquity. In ancient times, a soldier's horse might be sacrificed to accompany the fallen soldier in the next world. Hence the riderless horse would be part of the funeral procession symbolizing that the soldier would no longer ride on this side of life. In the US today, veterans are entitled to military honors that include the presentation of a folded flag and playing of *Taps* as well as the presence of uniformed military personnel.

War memorials also have a history. While originally memorials such as the Arc de Triomphe in Paris or London's Nelson's Column were built to commemorate victories, it soon became common to develop memorials that noted the sacrifice that war demanded. During the Civil War, for example, many towns dedicated memorials to commemorate their local loss. After World War I, there was some controversy over the development of "living memorials" such as Soldier Field, the home of the Chicago Bears, or Veterans Stadium, a multipurpose stadium in Philadelphia. In these cases, civic auditoriums, parks, libraries, or other community structures were built to serve the community while honoring the military. Far more controversial was a movement that emerged in France following the First World War where "pacifist" memorials were erected to the widows and orphans devastated by the losses of war. French soldiers were ordered to turn their heads when marching past such memorials.

Veterans cemeteries also date back to the Civil War. Prior to that, soldiers were often buried at the site of the battle, transported back home to be buried by the family, or interred at the military post. Given the high death toll of the Civil War, Congress created national cemeteries to honor those who had sacrificed their lives for the Union.

Sacred space and sacred ceremonies have long been part of the ways that we have dealt both with death in general and military deaths in particular. This chapter explores the ways that such sacred ceremonies and space can facilitate the grief of survivors, suggesting ways that such value may be enhanced when a veteran dies.

The Therapeutic Value of Funerals

Funeral rituals are a cultural universal since they offer so many therapeutic benefits (Rando, 1984). They are *rites of passage* that offer a ritualized marking of a change of status. In this case, funerals mark the transition between life and death. As such, they offer a symbolic vehicle that marks the death and allows the final disposition of remains.

Some of the benefits of funerals are psychological. First, funerals confirm the reality of death. One of the initial reactions to grief is often shock and disbelief.

This is especially true when a death is sudden, unexpected, and traumatic. Presence at a funeral, viewing the body, and hearing the condolences of others offer a constant reminder of the reality of the loss.

A second psychological benefit is that the funeral allows survivors to share memories and process feelings and reactions. In the community of family and friends, survivors have opportunities for emotional release and ventilation. This is critical in a number of ways. The funeral remains a vehicle where emotions can be openly expressed, allowing a catharsis. In addition, mourners can reminisce and share memories. The sharing of memories provides occasion to shape an image of the deceased as stories are remembered and discussed among the community. Both the expression of emotions and the recollection of memories are essential elements of the grieving process as they allow survivors to process the pain of the loss and forge an ongoing relationship with the deceased based on memory (Worden, 2008).

A final psychological benefit of the funeral is that the funeral allows the survivors to "do something" at an otherwise disorganized time. Participation in ritual allows symbolic mastery of the death. This can especially valuable in cases where the death was sudden or unexpected (Doka, 1984).

In addition to these psychological benefits, there are social benefits as well. One of the major benefits is that funerals offer an opportunity for the community to gather and offer support. This is critical in so many ways. It reaffirms that the community grieves together. This is especially important as the presence of caring others reaffirms that mourners are not alone as they cope with their grief.

Moreover, in the gathering of the funeral, there is sharing of stories, memories, and reminiscences. This sharing allows the mourners to make sense of the deceased's life, offering a sense that this life had value and meaning. This too is an essential aspect of the mourning process.

There is an additional social benefit as well. Often in the period of illness prior to the death, those in the intimate circle have been absorbed in caregiving, and may have been socially isolated. The funeral then serves to reintegrate them in their social circle by reaffirming ties, reestablishing social relationships, and publically reiterating the change in the mourners' status.

Funerals are spiritually significant. They offer an opportunity to provide a spiritual or philosophical interpretation of the death, contributing to meaning making. Funerals essentially provide a way to reflect on the meaning of this death within the community's philosophical or spiritual framework. The funeral itself, through familiar rituals, provides a sense of comfort and continuity even in times of insecurity and unknown change. It evokes the image of larger community that transcends the present and the promise of a continuing bond, however that might be interpreted within a given spirituality or philosophy. For members of a faith community, the funeral energizes that community to minister to the mourner.

Some of these benefits accrue to the group as a whole. Funerals allow the community to gather together showing both solidarity and support to the other mourners, and offer the promise that even with this death, the community survives. It allows the community to share memories and reminiscences. Finally, funerals help reconstruct both the meaning of the death and the nature of the continuing bond to the community as a whole.

Enhancing the Value of Funeral Rituals

While funeral rituals can be exceedingly therapeutic, there is much that can be done to even enhance the salutary significance of the rite. Early evidence has emphasized the value of planning and participating in funeral ceremonies (Doka, 1984). There are numerous opportunities and ways that this can be done. Family members can serve as pallbearers, readers, and eulogists. Depending on the religious service, such as in liturgical churches such as Anglican, Lutheran, and Roman Catholic, there may be other possibilities to participate. Adolescents may be employed as crucifers, acolytes, or altar boys. Even younger children can participate, perhaps handing out programs.

There is also a wide range of ways to personalize the funeral. Memory boards, photograph displays, and media presentations can highlight the life of the deceased, reaffirming the meaning and significance of life. Eulogies, personally selected music, and readers also enhance the individual quality of the rite.

Planning and participation can be especially therapeutic for instrumental grievers. Instrumental grievers are those who experience and express grief in more cognitive and physical ways (Doka and Martin, 2010). Since instrumental grievers often act on their grief, participation in both planning and conducting the funeral ritual can be very helpful. The style of grieving that an individual adapts is dependent on a variety of factors such as gender expectations, cultural norms, individual temperament, and socialization experiences. Persons who have experienced military culture may be more inclined to respond to grief in an instrumental way.

It is important to recognize two aspects of contemporary funerals. The first is that most individuals have multiple identities. That means that people generally only know one aspect of the deceased's life, as co-worker, family member, or neighbor. The funeral then may be the first time they see other facets of the deceased's life. Having multiple eulogists who can address these different aspects of a person can facilitate this process. In addition, it may be valuable to explain reasons that given readings or music are employed as only some of the participants may really understand the significance.

A number of years ago, a friend died in middle age after a dehabilitating disease. Prior to the illness, he was an engineer. However, his avocation was playing bluegrass music in a local band. They regularly played an open-air gig, provided the weather cooperated. Because their concert was always dependent on the weather, they began each set with a bluegrass rendition of *We'll Sing in the Sunshine*. When he learned of his diagnosis, he told his wife, "We learned to sing in the sunshine, now we will have to learn to sing in the rain." *Singing in the Rain* was the closing "hymn" of his funeral service. Yet the story needed to be told as only part of the audience would have appreciated the significance of the song.

A second factor relates to the diversity of cultural and spiritual backgrounds among participants in the funeral ritual. Few participants are likely to share the same cultural and spiritual roots, so there may be a need for cultural and spiritual translation, explaining what is occurring to those of different cultural or spiritual traditions.

The presence of military honors incorporated into the funeral service can be very therapeutic. Military honors are the right of every veteran honorably discharged from service. Military honors enhance the funeral ritual. These honors include the participation of two or more uniformed military personnel, the playing of *Taps*, and the folding and presentation of a burial flag. These honors reaffirm the service of the veteran, adding to a sense that the veteran's life had significance and meaning.

Sacred Space

The veteran also has the right to be buried in a veteran's cemetery. This too can reaffirm the meaning of the veteran's life in a number of ways. First, the presence of the veteran's remains in a space where other veterans are interred affirms that the veteran was a part of a larger enterprise, and is a reminder of the shared sacrifice. Second, it confirms the national gratitude for and recognition of service. Third, veterans cemeteries are often settings for other rituals marking, for example, Veterans and Memorial Day. These additional rites add significance and mark natural surges within the grief process.

Even if the family does not choose to bury the veteran in a veteran ceremony it is still important to have some sacred space to remember the deceased. One of the great values of cemeteries or memorial parks is that they allow families opportunities to visit a site on appropriate days and to conduct their own rituals; leaving flowers, for example, on special times such as holidays, birthdays, or meaningful anniversaries. Veterans memorials can serve as alternate or complementary locations for such ceremonies.

The Value of Therapeutic Ritual

While funeral rituals can be highly therapeutic, they are, by nature, limited; the funeral takes place in the immediate aftermath of the death. Grief, however, is an ongoing process. The presence of other rituals throughout the grieving process, whether anniversary services or masses, patriotic rituals, or private family rituals, can mark other points in the journey of grief.

Therapeutic rituals can also be utilized. Therapeutic rituals are rituals that are incorporated within the therapeutic or counseling process. Such rituals focus on specific therapeutic goals and reaffirm specific therapeutic messages (Doka and Martin, 2010). Such rituals may be performed by individuals or larger groups such as the intimate network of survivors. They can be a bridge to an individual's culture or spirituality by incorporating elements of that culture, faith, or philosophy into the rite.

Therapeutic rituals have a specific message. One such message may be one of continuity. *Rituals of continuity* reaffirm a continuing bond with the deceased, recognition that the relationship is retained even in death. In many ways, these are relatively common rituals that may be undertaken in a wide variety of settings. Participation in an anniversary ritual, toasting a deceased individual on a birthday, or lighting a candle are all examples of such a ritual. Veterans and Memorial Day both provide a public ritual where the value of service and sacrifice and the continuing bond are nationally affirmed.

Rituals of transition are designed to indicate movement within the process of grief. In one such ritual, a young adolescent idolized his deceased grandfather, a

Vietnam veteran. He even kept his grandfather's photograph on his night table. His grandmother began to date again, about 18 months after his grandfather's death. At first the boy was resistant and resentful of both his grandmother and her new beau. With some encouragement from his own parents and assistance from his school counselor, he became more accepting of the relationship. After his grandmother's remarriage, he asked for a photograph of his new grandfather. He placed it in a frame that held two photographs, one for each grandfather, signifying his acceptance of this new relationship in his life.

Rituals of reconciliation allow mourners to finish business. Such rituals can permit the mourner to give or to receive forgiveness. Often the Vietnam Veterans Memorial in Washington, DC, offers a space for such rituals. In one, an unknown medic left a note attached to a name on the wall. "I want you to know, I did everything possible to save you. You're here. It was not enough. I'm sorry."

Rituals of affirmation complement rituals of reconciliation. Here the message is to affirm the deceased. A ritual of affirmation fundamentally thanks the deceased for their contributions. In one such ritual, an elderly wife of a veteran ceremoniously passed on to her adult children the medals their deceased father had won for service in the Korean War. To her it was important to have a ritual where she could explain the significance of her husband's service to her children, honoring his memory and affirming the meaningfulness of his life.

In creating therapeutic rituals, a few principles should be employed. First, the ritual should emerge from the narrative. Each ritual has to be individually constructed, arising from the client's individual story. There is no template for any therapeutic ritual. Second, the ritual should include tangible objects that also have symbolic significance. Rituals revolve around objects; they offer a focal point for the rite. The medals, photograph, or letter remind participants of the qualities and message they wish to confer in the ceremony.

Rituals also have to be planned and processed, and the planning needs to be both therapeutic and practical. From a therapeutic context, the counselor should ask questions clarifying the message of the ritual and affirming the significance of the acts and objects that will comprise the rite. The client may wish to consider if this is a private or public ceremony as well as if there may be others who will participate or witness the event. There may need to be practical issues that have to be considered. For example, in the ritual of affirmation described earlier, the mother was asking her sons and their families to be part of this ritual. This led to other questions such as the timing of the ritual, as well as details as to whether she would serve a meal to the family, what the menu would be, and what accommodation would be made for a granddaughter coming from a distance.

The counselor also needs to process the ritual with the client following the experience. *How did the client react during the rite? Did the ritual accomplish the client's goals and expectations? What worked well? What might have been done differently? Are there other things the client needs to do?*

Finally, in preparing a ritual, there are lessons to be learned from faith communities. Rituals all take on a special character when they are encased in the primal elements of fire (candles), wind (music or chimes), water, and soil (flowers).

As this chapter began, it was noted that rituals began far back in antiquity. Long before writing, long before the domestication of plants and animals, long before the emergence of settled communities, our ancient ancestors acknowledged the power and importance of ritual. It is a lesson that should never be lost or forgotten.

Kenneth J. Doka, PhD, MDiv, is a professor of gerontology at the Graduate School of The College of New Rochelle and senior consultant to the Hospice Foundation of America. Dr. Doka serves as editor of HFA's Living with Grief *book series, its* Journeys *newsletter, and numerous other books and publications. Dr. Doka has served as a panelist on HFA's* Living with Grief ® *video programs for 20 years. He is a past president of the Association for Death Education and Counseling (ADEC) and received an award for Outstanding Contributions in the field of Death Education. He is a member and past chair of the International Work Group on Death, Dying and Bereavement. In 2006, Dr. Doka was grandfathered in as a mental health counselor under New York's first state licensure of counselors. Dr. Doka is an ordained Lutheran minister.*

REFERENCES

Doka, K.J. (1984). Expectation of death, participation in planning funeral rituals and grief adjustment. *Omega: Journal of Death and Dying, 15,* 119-130.

Doka, K.J., & Martin, T.L. (2010). *Grieving beyond gender: Understanding the ways men and women mourn.* New York, NY: Routledge.

Rando, T.A. (1984). *Grief, dying and death: Clinical interventions for caregivers.* Champaign, IL: Research Press.

Worden, J.W. (2008). *Grief counseling and grief therapy: A handbook for the mental health practitioner* (4th Ed.). New York, NY: Springer.

CHAPTER 16

Profaning the Sacred: The Disruption of Military Funerals

Kenneth J. Doka

E ven in times of contentious conflicts, the sacrifices made by military personnel were generally acknowledged by those who might protest the war. In most recent wars, even enemies showed respect for the fallen on both sides. Historically, armies often called a truce to respectfully remove the bodies of fallen comrades.

This respect, historically extended to fallen soldiers, was challenged in 2005 when Fred Phelps and members of his Westboro Baptist Church, a small fringe group of inter-related families in Topeka, KS, began to conduct protests at the funerals of soldiers who had died in Afghanistan and Iraq. Phelps' underlying rationale behind these protests was that these deaths were God's punishment to America for tolerating homosexuality. Prior to picketing military deaths, members of the Westboro Baptist Church picketed the funerals of gay individuals and those who had died of AIDS-related illnesses, as well as politicians and celebrities known to be sympathetic to the lesbian, gay, bisexual, and transgender (LGBT) community. At military funerals, Phelps' band of protestors would display signs that read "God hates fags" and "Thank God for dead soldiers," even though none of the deceased had ever identified as gay.

The actions of the Westboro Baptist Church have generated considerable reactions. A number of states have passed laws prohibiting picketing within certain distance from funeral homes or funeral services. The U.S. Congress passed, and President G.W. Bush signed, the *Respect for American Fallen Heroes Act* that prohibits picketing within 300 feet of a national cemetery within an hour prior to or after a funeral. In addition to these legal endeavors, individuals have found a number of ways to respond to the disruption of military funerals by the Westboro Baptist Church. A motorcycle group called the Patriot Guard

Riders, consisting primarily of veterans, will attend the funerals of veterans at the request of the deceased family. Their attendance both shows support and drowns out the comments of the protestors by the roaring of their engines. In other cases, members of the community create human walls to shield mourners from the signs and taunts of church members.

Albert Snyder, the parent of a deceased veteran, sued Phelps and the group for intentional infliction of emotional distress along with other issues. Snyder won a significant judgment of close to 11 million dollars in a lower court. The decision was overturned by the U.S. Supreme Court in 2011 on the basis that, however odious, the actions of the Westboro Baptist Church were protected by the First Amendment.

Westboro's actions probably have had mixed impact on the funerals of veterans. On one hand, opposition to the stance of this church from all ends of the political spectrum has often led to an outpouring of community support. On the other hand, the anxiety generated by the protest as the disruption of somber ceremony no doubt complicates the grief of survivors. Certainly even with the support of a wide spectrum of the community, families had to endure public conflict and controversy in what should be a private opportunity for family and friends to come together to grieve their loss.

Editor's Note: In the interest of full disclosure, Dr. Kenneth J. Doka (author) was called as an expert witness in Snyder v. Phelps to address the deleterious effects of the disruption of funerals on the grief of survivors.

CHAPTER 17

Serving the Bereavement Needs of Veterans and Their Families

Patricia McGuire

Veterans and their families need the same things non-veterans and their families need when a loss is experienced: comfort, sympathy, emotional support of friends and family, knowledge, coping skills, time, and healing. But the military culture can create special grief needs as well.

Stoicism, while a needed quality for an operative military, can be a hindrance in grief. Stoicism may cause grief to be hidden by a silent or angry facade, cavalier humor, an attitude of bravado, or an "I'm fine" wall of denial. Stoicism not only affects veterans, it can affect whole family systems. One woman spoke of her friend who was married to a career Marine. She described the woman's stoicism: "She is as much a Marine as he is. When her mother died, she was expected to grieve quickly and return to normal functioning in short order. She did." Twenty years later, however, her mother's death was reactivated when her husband died. This time, she was given permission and encouragement to grieve and to take the time she needed to grieve both of these losses. She did.

In addition to stoicism, "career-military" family systems may present special considerations. The family may have lived in numerous places for short periods of time, and this impacts family in several different ways. For example, at one veteran's deathbed, his adult daughter identified for the first time where her bitterness for her father had begun: "It was the five different first grades I went to." Since this veteran was dying in a Veterans Administration (VA) hospice and the staff had been trained in veteran-specific issues, his daughter made this discovery as part of her anticipatory grief. She had the opportunity to work through this issue and the wall it had created before her father died. The clinician acknowledged the patriotism and sacrifice that her entire family had made, which allowed the daughter to change her relationship to her past. This change helped her let go of some of her anger and open up to her father in a new way. Her grief after his death was facilitated by acknowledging the ways that this early loss affected her life and her perception of her father, which helped her deal with those losses prior to her father's death.

Another issue which may arise with career-military families is that when there is a death or major loss, the family may find themselves far away from their family and support system. Because military families have not established roots, there may not be a network of support that facilitates effective grieving. On the other hand, because of these frequent moves, families of veterans may readily reach out for support because they have learned how to ask for help and form new bonds quickly. A Greek war bride from WWII cried at her husband's death bed: "I have no family, what am I going to do?" The staff anticipated the possibility of complicated grief due to lack of support. An hour later, however, she was found in the hospice kitchen, with five lifelong friends from the Officers' Wives Club. It was every bit a supportive family, just a different kind. Conversely a young Vietnamese wife who barely spoke English said: "We did everything together. We are each other's world." This veteran's isolation excluded everyone except his wife, leaving her unprepared for his death. She was at high risk for complications of grief and required extensive support to find her way materially and emotionally after his death.

Consider a third young American bride living in Germany while her husband served in Afghanistan. He was due to return in time for the birth of their first child. Unfortunately, the young woman went into labor early and their child was delivered stillborn. She was far from home, family, and anything familiar as she struggled with her overwhelming grief. Her husband returned to her as soon as possible, which in this case was a week later. He was grieving the loss of their child, feeling like he deserted his platoon and struggling with symptoms of Posttraumatic Stress Disorder (PTSD). She was grieving the loss of their baby, the loss of innocence as she saw the changes in her husband, and experiencing changes in her body. This couple required intensive support as they faced their changed world. Their return to home was delayed due to legal issues related to transporting their child's remains from one country to another so the priority was to assist their parents to travel to them. This whole family system may need extensive support due to the complexity of the situation.

In her book, *Peace at Last: Stories of Hope and Healing for Veterans and Their Families*, Deborah Grassman (2009) explores the impact of military service on veterans at the end of life. She offers insight into some of the possible effects of combat on veterans and their families. Providing the book for family members to read helps them better understand the military influence on their loved one, their family, and themselves. This enhanced understanding can facilitate peaceful life closure and more effective grief recovery.

Veterans may gain a deeper appreciation of life by surviving combat and recognizing each day as a gift. Others may superficially integrate their experiences and carry on with their pre-war lives after returning from war. A third group may be changed by their combat experience and be unable to effectively cope. These latter two groups' coping styles may adversely affect the family. Veterans in the last category may have struggled for years with bouts of depression, anger, nightmares, or from being overly protective or controlling. The veteran may have coped by using drugs and alcohol, or might have isolated himself in order to feel safe. Families living in this environment may have been abandoned, abused, or developed dysfunctional coping mechanisms to deal with these behaviors. This kind of lifestyle might precipitate divorce, creating multiple families by the time the veteran comes to the end of life. A common saying among Vietnam vets that overly simplifies this issue is, "Most veterans with PTSD have been married three times." There may be three different sets of children at a veteran's death bed. Perhaps their first family was abandoned when the veteran first returned home from war and he was unable to reconnect with them. These children may be angry. When the veteran remarried and started a second family, these children may have lived with abuse, drugs and alcohol, and developed dysfunctional coping mechanisms. After a second divorce, the veteran may have gotten into an addiction recovery program, as well as received help for his PTSD. A third marriage is often to someone who already has children. These children may reap the benefit of the veteran's recovery and think their stepfather is very special. Imagine this veteran's death bed with all of these family members present. Providing support for all of these family members with a wide range of forgiveness, estrangement, and anger issues creates a highly charged environment for needed therapeutic work. Clinicians should strive to keep their hearts open to all of these different family members and recognize each of the particular losses and relationships with this veteran, in order to help facilitate some resolution. The past cannot be changed, but new understanding can help to change their relationships to the past.

When there are multiple families, judgments about one another are often passed. Guilt, shame, and blame are often the fuel that has been used to avoid the pain of the underlying loss of healthy relationships. This can negatively impact decisions that need to be made as the veteran is approaching the end of life. For example, the person who is legally able to make the decisions for the veteran may be someone from whom the veteran has been estranged. The current significant others of the veteran may find themselves disenfranchised at the time of the death, funeral, and burial. Another common contention after the death of a veteran with this kind of multiple-family constellation is: "Who gets the flag?" There is one flag provided for each veteran, yet there may be more than one person who feels that they deserve it. In these situations, it can be helpful to work with the VA's office of Decedent Affairs, also known as Details Clerk, to arrange for the provision of more than one flag.

Presentation of the flag in a respectful manner is of the utmost importance. Because many families today choose cremation, there may or may not be a funeral or memorial. In these cases there is not a formal presentation of the tri-corner flag to the next of kin. One VA nurse saw a family leaving the hospice unit after their loved one's death with a flag in a small rectangular box. He was upset by this "indignity" and called the team together to find a way to correct it. The solution was found when the Korean War Veterans Service Organization (VSO) agreed to use this need as an opportunity. The VSO provided education to a local Boy Scout troop about proper flag etiquette and flag folding. The Boy Scouts now meet bi-monthly with the VSO to fold flags. Together, they have maintained a supply of folded flags for that VA facility. The flag is now formally presented in a dignified way to the family by the Decedent Affairs Clerk.

Other family members might have anger or bitterness about their veteran not getting a medal, service-connected disability, or pension. These feelings can interfere with effective grieving: "Dad was wounded in combat and he never received his Purple Heart. They lost his records." This veteran and his entire family had chafed over this injustice for many years. After his father's death, one son doggedly pursued his father's records until the Purple Heart was awarded posthumously. This act helped the family begin to move through their grief. In a similar situation in which the Purple Heart could not be obtained, a VA hospice nurse practitioner made a "purple heart," ceremonially pinning it on the veteran while citing the heroic deeds that he had done. The bereaved family survey subsequently identified this act as extremely meaningful.

If PTSD is identified for the first time as a veteran is dying, the impact on family needs to be factored into their bereavement needs. Some family members feel relief: "I'm so glad to know it has a name. I knew something was wrong but I didn't know what. Now this makes sense." Other family members might feel guilty: "I wish I would've realized this sooner, I would have_____ (listened more carefully, gotten him help, been more patient and understanding, etc.)" (NHPCO VAC, 2012).

If the veteran had PTSD, physical or mental disability, or long-term illness prior to the death, the family member may be exhausted from providing care; they may not have the energy to grieve. In her book *Chronic Sorrow: A Living Loss*, Louise Roos (2002) writes about "significant losses with no foreseeable end" in the context of children with disabilities. Veterans and their families may share a similar experience. This may lead to frequent periods of sadness with no stable periods to allow time for grief and adjustment.

The family may have financial concerns near the end of life. For example, if the family has been supported by the veteran's disability check, they may want extensive futile care because they do not know how they will survive without the veteran's check. They may have provided care for the veteran for years and thus been unable to maintain work outside the home. It is important for the clinician to acknowledge the reality of this practical consideration and recognize that the family's questions about money may not indicate a lack of love, but instead may be a first step in providing the practical groundwork for their future welfare and their ability to grieve. Providing social work services can help the family with financial strategies and resources. The veteran may also be concerned about the financial plight of their family after he or she dies. This concern might cause the veteran to fight death so the disability check continues. One veteran lived for 40 years as a quadriplegic in a VA nursing home. He said, "My job is to stay alive as long as I can so my wife will have the money to raise our kids." When he died, his family spoke of "growing up at the VA," and there were as many staff mourners as family at the memorial service. Many such families have provided care and support for their loved one for years with little or no recognition. Acknowledgment of their patriotism and a word of gratitude for the sacrifices they have made may bring tears to their eyes. Those tears often represent the internal healing that is taking place. One VA recognizes the family members who have been caring for veterans by pinning them with a small patriotic angel dressed in red, white, and blue. The family is thanked for their sacrifices and service to America by providing care and support to their veteran. A small card is given to them so they will remember the meaning behind the pinning. The card reads: "Caregivers are important too! Because we know you have also paid a price for our freedom, we honor you with this pin. It's our way of acknowledging the many ways you've been impacted by the military and also the many ways you have provided care to our veteran. We are grateful."

Caregivers are 93% female. Most caregivers are spouses (72%) and parents(12%) (National Alliance for Caregiving, 2012). Today, there are more services for family caregivers than ever before. All VA medical centers now have Caregiver Support Coordinators at all VA medical centers (Johnson, 2012). They are experts on caregiver issues and are knowledgeable about VA and non-VA resources. They manage a menu of options to support veterans including in-home care service, respite care, needed equipment, home and automobile modification, peer support, and caregiver support groups. The VA also runs an interactive website for caregivers (www.caregiver.va.gov). The Primary Family Caregiver Benefits include a stipend (post-9/11) paid directly to the caregiver, which is centrally funded and managed. The caregiver may be eligible for health insurance through CHAMPVA (a health benefits program through VA), travel, lodging and mental health services through VA or by contract. This kind of support allows veterans and their families to have more time and energy for their bereavement and emotional needs.

In addition to needing support when a veteran is facing illness and death, family members may also need help in understanding a veteran's response to loss. A veteran's inability to grieve someone's death might be due to their fear of unresolved grief from comrades who died in combat, and this fear can sometimes cause the veteran to detach from grief. This was true for a veteran and father of four whose youngest son was killed in a hit-and-run motor vehicle accident. The veteran went through the formalities of identifying the body, arranging the funeral, and receiving the outpouring of support from his community; yet he remained impassive throughout the process. His wife and family were appalled at his lack of emotion. When the veteran came in for counseling, he reported being in Vietnam 40 years earlier and being on a convoy. One of the trucks in the convoy hit a young Vietnamese boy. It was a dangerous area and they were under orders not to stop. This veteran was devastated by seeing this innocent boy left presumably dead and unattended. When his own son died in a similar manner, he could not allow himself to feel the grief for his own son until he had acknowledged the loss and grief of the parents of the Vietnamese boy. The latter was the focus of the bereavement intervention.

Another young soldier serving in Iraq was notified of his grandfather's death; the Red Cross was prepared to bring him home for the funeral. The soldier declined to leave his troop, and the family was very upset with his decision. The bereavement counselor discussed with the family their son's need for stoicism so he could face war every day. If he came home for the funeral, he may have felt that he had deserted his troop. He could also be opening himself up to an emotional bungee jump, bouncing from his feelings of his grandfather's loss which could also trigger grief over deaths he was seeing in war, only to have to go right back into war two weeks later. Thus, the bereavement intervention did not focus on trying to convince the grandson of the need to return home, but rather on helping the family choose to validate the young soldier's choice. Intervention also focused on planning a family gathering when the young soldier was home again and emotionally able to participate in working through his grief for both his grandfather and his fallen comrades.

SUPPORTING VETERAN GRIEF

As part of a focus on comprehensive care, the VA identifies unresolved bereavement needs of veterans when they are being treated for physical and mental health issues, homelessness, substance abuse, and PTSD. These needs can best be addressed by a clinician who has been sensitized to the special needs of veterans. In 2003, *Wounded Warriors: Their Last Battle*, a PowerPoint presentation developed by Deborah Grassman, was produced by the National Hospice and Palliative Care Organization (NHPCO) and distributed widely throughout both the hospice and VA communities. Her presentation sensitizes clinicians, veterans, and their families to issues that may otherwise be overlooked or misunderstood. The same stoicism that allows veterans to be the helpers of the world may prevent them from reaching out for help or support. Messages of "big boys and girls don't cry" were learned as children and reinforced in the military. This message needs to be reframed by clinicians. When a veteran is talking about the pain of loss and attempting to hold back the tears, they can be reminded of the courage it takes to allow their feelings to show. It may be helpful to sit beside rather than in front of the veteran to allow emotional privacy. Alternatively, the clinician might bow their head and sit quietly when tears escape from behind a stoic wall. Clinicians can let veterans know that tears are a normal reaction to pain and are welcome. One counselor has a picture of a face with a beautiful tear running down it. The picture is referenced with veterans who struggle to externalize tears, and acts as a reminder of the beauty of grief expressed. Another counselor has a prescription pad and "prescribes" crying in the shower, in the car, or wherever the veteran feels safe. Some veterans are more comfortable with humor and respond well to being told that the counselor gets a bonus if they cry. Everyone grieves in their own way, so there are not always tears. The gender differences between men and women have been studied for years and many men are more likely to express their grief by doing something active, such as planting a tree, building a memorial, or organizing a fundraiser for a needy veteran family. Tears may or may not be part of their grief journey (Doka and Martin, 2010; Golden, 2010).

In caring for veterans with PTSD, it is important to know that they may not trust easily. Initial efforts by clinicians need to focus on gaining their trust. This can make something as simple as scheduling an appointment difficult. For example, when a veteran is identified for bereavement counseling, a telephone call is used to make contact. Not unusually, there is no answer and a message is left encouraging a call back. When this is unsuccessful, a second call is made and again a message is left. If the call is not returned, a condolence note is mailed to the home. Persistence often pays off at this point and the veteran may reconnoiter and peek into the bereavement office a few times. If the counselor passes muster and seems trustworthy, the veteran will schedule an appointment to address his or her grief issues. A basic premise of passing muster is the clinician's understanding that "we serve those who first served us." Veterans need to know that clinicians are aware that veterans are trained warriors; they need to know that clinicians value their service and recognize that freedom is not free.

These issues may also be apparent when a veteran is diagnosed with a terminal disease. The veteran may not want anyone "to see me weak." They may go so far as to say, "When I can't take care of myself, I'll just go off into the woods to die." One such veteran received interventions during his several admissions to the hospital during his illness. The clinician's interventions focused on encouraging him to be a gracious receiver. He was educated about Dame Cicely Saunders, founder of the modern hospice movement around the world, and what she said at a conference a few years before her death. Using a wheelchair for ambulation, she stated, "I used to think that being a giver was the most important thing. Now that I need help myself, I realize that being a gracious receiver is the most important thing." He was encouraged to see how helpful his gracious receiving could be for him and for his comrades.

As his illness progressed, he was able to make healthier decisions about his care. The veteran allowed his friends in the "Vietnam Brotherhood" to participate in his care and ultimately his death. Many of these men had only witnessed violent or mutilating deaths in the past. In combat there was no time to mourn the deaths of comrades. This veteran made a courageous choice to allow the brotherhood to come together as a group to grieve while they provided care and support to their dying comrade. They were dressed in their Vietnam Brotherhood jackets; many had long hair, ponytails, and tattoos. Although their tough exteriors were intimidating, they provided tender physical comfort by repositioning the veteran, giving him drinks of water and food, and even participating in circles of prayer. By relying on their camaraderie and overcoming their fear of vulnerability, they created a dignified death for their friend and a new concept about death for themselves.

The Commander of a local chapter of the Korean War Veterans Service Organization (VSO) was asked about the impact of combat on the members. His eyes clouded over: "We all have PTSD to some degree. It's just a matter of what we do with it." He spoke of some members who self-medicated with alcohol, but of many others who channeled their pain into contributing to the community. Honor guards are one of the services this chapter provides. They are frequently at the local VA cemetery to honor their newly fallen comrades by providing military honors, an interment ceremony, and the presentation of the flag to the next of kin. He acknowledged that when he participates in these events, he is attending to his own bereavement needs by honoring the buddies he lost in service so long ago.

As many as 30,000 veterans live in State Veteran Homes and there are many other long-term care facilities caring for veterans. These settings can provide an opportunity to address unresolved grief from fallen comrades decades earlier.

One State Veterans Home in Ohio provides such a service. The team of clinicians prepares a sacred space in the front of a large meeting room. A long table holds the American flag and other patriotic symbols. Veterans are encouraged to think in advance about a fallen comrade they might want to honor during the ceremony. As they gather, patriotic music plays and the lights are lowered to accent the importance of the occasion. At the entrance, there are small rocks for each veteran to select and take with them to their seats. The ceremony is opened by the chaplain with a prayer of remembrance for all those who had died, as well as those who are still in the beds next to them. The social worker does a guided imagery with the veterans, taking them into those deep parts of themselves where they store their feelings. Then soothing music is played as they are invited to write the name of the person they wish to honor on the rock they are holding. Some of the veterans request additional rocks because the ceremony causes other unresolved losses to the surface. The tasks of dying healed (Forgive me, I forgive you, I love you, Thank you, Goodbye), from Ira Byock's book *Dying Well* (1997), may be read to offer the option of completing any unfinished business. The veterans are encouraged to say in their hearts whatever they need to say to the person. Then one by one, each veteran carries his or her rock forward, placing it on the sacred space. Staff caregivers are also encouraged to participate and include those veterans they've cared for whom they wish to remember. A closing blessing offers hope for the future. The veterans are told that these rocks would remain in the sacred space for one month; the veterans would be later invited back to transport the rocks to an outdoor area of remembrance that would remain accessible to them. Singing of patriotic songs closes the ceremony. At each ceremony, there are many tears as these veterans allow themselves to confront their losses and begin moving through them.

The value of rituals cannot be underestimated, especially because ritual has been a successful aspect of military culture throughout the years. An effective ritual consists of three stages: separation, transition, and integration. The separation phase acknowledges the problem. In the above example, this was done with the chaplain's prayer and the guided imagery; both validated the loss that each veteran experienced. The transition phase focuses on educating participants in how to proceed with this change and loss. In the ceremony with the rocks, this was done by the bereavement counselor who spoke about the value of grief, encouraging them to re-think their stoic stances. The value of completing "unfinished business" with Byock's five tasks was provided. The last phase, integration, was accomplished by encouraging the veterans to let go of what was and open up to a new normal. This was done by physically placing their rocks in the sacred place, knowing that their comrade's memories would continue with them. The integrative process would continue as the veterans would visit the outdoor area of remembrance whenever they wanted.

Throughout the United States, there are memorials and ceremonies taking place nearly every day. These can be healing to both veterans and their families. Most VA Medical Centers offer memorial services honoring the veterans who died in their facility annually. These services should be formatted in a ritualized ceremony that acknowledges and promotes effective grieving and the ceremony should have a military context. Many VAs provide bereavement ceremonies or events to provide support for the veterans and their families for Memorial Day, Veterans Day, Fourth of July, and other holidays. Including veterans and their families in these events can be very helpful with their grief.

Active-duty deaths

The military culture influences both veterans and their families. They may face issues that do not impact the general population. This is also true of veterans and families of loved ones dying on active duty; however, hospice services are not provided to families prior to an active military death. Bereavement care to the surviving family members should follow the above guidelines coupled with standard bereavement guidelines that focus on sudden and violent death.

There are two organizations that are uniquely equipped to provide bereavement counseling and support to active duty personnel, their families, and extended families: Vet Centers and Tragedy Assistance Program for Survivors (TAPS). Vet Centers provide individual, group, and family counseling to all veterans who served in any combat zone. Services are also available for their family members. TAPS is a national non-profit organization that offers extensive peer-to-peer support and education about traumatic death and the active duty military's specific grief needs. Some hospices partner with these agencies to provide services. Other hospices partner with the Red Cross to offer bereavement services for active military deaths. Hospice staff receive specialized training in order to perform this task.

CONCLUSION

Supporting veterans in grief and loss is essential, but servicemen and women's military training can hamper this process. Stoic grief sometimes postpones reacting and responding to losses. When the stoic facade begins to crumble, losses accumulated over a lifetime may surface. Families of veterans may also have special needs in grief. The fallout of war often infiltrates families and causes scars and divisions which require special attention. Clinicians need to continue to learn how to better serve those who first served us.

Editor's Note: The contents of this paper do not represent the views of the Department of Veterans Affairs or the United States Government.

Patricia McGuire, *RN, BSN, CT, is the Bereavement Coordinator of the Bay Pines VA Healthcare System. Over the past 16 years, first as a hospice nurse, and then 12 years as bereavement coordinator, she has worked with thousands of veterans and their families as they navigate their grief.*

REFERENCES

Byock, I. (1997). *Dying well: Peace and possibilities at end of life*. New York, NY: Riverhead Books.

Doka, K. J., & Martin, T. (2010). *Grieving beyond gender: Understanding the ways men and women mourn* (rev. ed.). New York, NY: Routledge.

Golden, T. (2010). *Swallowed by a snake: The gift of the masculine side of healing*. Gaithersburg, MD: Golden Healing Publishing.

Grassman, D. (2009). *Peace at last: Stories of hope and healing for veterans and their families*. St. Petersburg, FL: Vandamere Press.

Johnson, N. (2012, September). *Caring for the Veteran caregiver*. PowerPoint Presentation at Northeast Florida Community Hospice conference, Jacksonville, FL.

National Alliance for Caregiving. (2012, December). Retrieved from http://www.caregiving.org

National Hospice and Palliative Care Organization. (Producer). (2003). *Wounded warriors: Their last battle* [PowerPoint presentation]. Available from http://www.wehonorveterans.org/

National Hospice and Palliative Care Organization's Veterans Advisory Council. (2012). *Wounded warriors: Their last battle/ facilitator's guide for grief work with veterans' families*. Alexandria, VA: Author.

Roos, Louise. (2002). *Chronic sorrow: A living loss*. New York, NY: Brunner-Routledge.

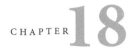

Combat Death: A Clinical Perspective

Jill Harrington-LaMorie with Betsy Beard

The blow that killed a soldier on the field...also sent waves of misery and desolation into a world of relatives and friends, who themselves became war's casualties. (Faust, 2008, p. 143)

In the last two centuries the United States has participated in 12 wars, both foreign and domestic. In its first 100 years of existence, more than 683,000 Americans lost their lives in American wars, with the Civil War accounting for 623,000 of that total (91.2%). In the next 100 years, a further 626,000 American service members died serving in two World Wars and other wars, with World War II representing 65% of that total.

When one man dies it's a tragedy. When thousands die it's a statistic. (Antonov-Ovseyenko, 1981, p. 278)

No matter the number of deceased each war may bring, every death is an individual, highly personal loss to relatives and friends of that service member who was killed in battle. That service member was someone's son, daughter, brother, sister, husband, wife, significant other, mother, father, grandchild, nephew, niece, friend, or comrade. The survivors' lives are indelibly altered by the notification that their service member has been killed in action. Combat death casualties do not end at the reportable number of deceased; they are magnified exponentially by those families and friends left in their wake.

The death of a close loved one is a universal human experience and is recognized as one of life's most difficult and distressing events. Additionally, when a family member dies in combat for the U.S. military, the common observation generally supported by anecdotal evidence is that combat death presents a burdensome grief with unique factors that can lead to complications

189

in bereavement for survivors. This, in turn, leads to challenges for clinicians and caregivers.

Combat death is familiar ground for Americans. We are a nation born out of revolution, and as long as there have been standing militia and armed forces in the US, there have been combat deaths. Surprisingly, there is a lack of empirical evidence on the impact on surviving families of those killed in action in the U.S. military and how best to help survivors (Harrington-LaMorie and McDevitt-Murphy, 2011). In general, surviving military families are a poorly understood and understudied population.

Given the young age of the deceased, the sudden and/or violent circumstances of death, and the young age of many of the survivors, as well as circumstantial factors unique to military death, very little is known about the risk and resilience factors of this vulnerable population and best therapeutic interventions for care. Our knowledge of bereavement and adaptation to loss in military families who have endured the combat death of a U.S. service member is principally anecdotal from observation and first-person accounts of survivors. In the past decade, there has been a growing body of literature on the dual influences of grief and trauma. Given that the US is a nation still at war, with service members being killed in action, there is an imminent need for research in this area.

For the purposes of this chapter, we will focus primarily on the impact of the death of a service member who has been killed as a result of hostile action during the wars in Iraq and Afghanistan. The impact to families of origin (parents and siblings) and families of procreation (spouses and children) will be explored. The goal of this chapter is to provide clinicians and caregivers a better understanding of demographics of the survivors, complicating military factors that impact survivors, and clinical issues.

DEMOGRAPHICS OF THE DECEASED AND THE SURVIVORS

Operation Enduring Freedom (OEF) and Operation Iraqi Freedom (OIF): The Wars in Afghanistan and Iraq

Approximately 1.4 million American military personnel have served on active status in the Armed Services (Army, Navy, Air Force, Marines, and Coast Guard) in all components (Active, Reserve, and National Guard), since the inception of the wars in Afghanistan in 2001 and Iraq in 2003 (DMDC, 2012).

Over the past decade, there have been more than 16,000 military deaths in active-duty status, with over one-third of these deaths attributed to the wars in Iraq and Afghanistan (DMDC, 2012). The overwhelming majority of military deaths on active status are sudden and/or violent in nature and involve the death of an adolescent or young adult. At the time this chapter was written, 6,630 American service members had died in Iraq and Afghanistan (DMDC, 2012) of which 5,211 were combat deaths. 26.2% of all military deaths have occurred in Iraq and 9.9% in Afghanistan (DMDC, 2012).

The largest demographic of deaths are of enlisted E1-E9 (89%), men (97%), between the ages of 18-30 (85%) (DMDC, 2012). The Department of Defense (DoD) categorizes conflict casualties with two broad categories: hostile (killed in action) and non-hostile (died in war zone). Hostile deaths may include deaths from enemy gunfire, improvised explosive devices (IEDs), torture, sniper fire, rocket-propelled grenades, suicide bombers, and air losses. In war, mass casualties often occur, with multiple service members killed at the same time, perhaps due to an aircraft being shot down or a vehicle being blown up. Non-hostile deaths include accidents, homicide, suicide, and illness.

All branches of the military (Army, Navy, Air Force, and Marines) have incurred casualties during combat, with the Army and Marine Corps suffering the highest numbers (DMDC, 2012). All three components (Active Duty, Reserve, and National Guard) have been affected. When a service member is killed in action, homicide is listed as the cause of death on the death certificate. Many survivors describe the same grief reactions of those of homicide survivors.

A snapshot of surviving families: OEF/OIF

Given the age (18-30) of the majority of casualties associated with the wars in Iraq and Afghanistan, the typical profile of a surviving family of a service member may include young parents (who may be young adults themselves), young siblings, a young spouse/adult partner, pediatric and adolescent children (some unborn), and a generally younger group of extended family members and friends.

Very little information is known about survivor demographics, except for information based on age and residence kept by the Department of Defense (DoD) and Department of Veteran's Affairs (VA) on surviving spouses and dependent children for the purpose of benefits. Family survivors reside in all 50 states and outside the continental US. Surviving spouses and children may choose to live closer to military bases after the death to utilize military benefits, although some choose to move where they find higher social support from family, friends, or new employment.

The "typical" Primary Next of Kin (PNOK) of a service member is a parent (if the service member is unmarried) or spouse (if the service member is married), while the "typical" Secondary Next of Kin (SNOK) can be a parent (if married) or sibling or other close relation (if unmarried). The military formally focuses its resources and support on the PNOK and SNOK listed by service members on their personnel paperwork. However, all who have felt an attachment to the service member can be either outwardly or silently grieving the loss. These disenfranchised grievers may include siblings, cousins, friends, stepparents, aunts, uncles, grandparents, fiancés, same-sex partners, ex-spouses, or others in a significant relationship. A vastly underrecognized population who are at risk for direct exposure to trauma and grief are fellow uniformed service members, especially those with whom they have served in combat.

Each service member who dies in combat impacts multiple micro, mezzo, and macro systems: the members of the unit in which they served; their immediate and extended families by whom they are survived; the casualty and mortuary affairs personnel who tend to their burial and remains; the death notification teams; military families living on posts or bases from which they are deployed; communities in which they have lived or been raised; the greater military community at large; and the American public. Providers of care should become aware of the multi-systematic impacts of trauma and how to best support the individual and collective grief of these communities (Zinner and Williams, 1999).

GRIEF AND TRAUMA

Death is a universal, natural part of the human experience (Worden, 2009). Grief is the normal, natural, necessary reaction to an overwhelming and distressing loss in life. It can affect every part of our being: mind, body, spirit, and social being. Grief is a highly individualized and subjective experience that allows us to let go of that which was and prepares us for that which is to come. Though the experience of grief is universal, the death of each individual person is experienced differently, in its own unique way and its own unique time. This is part of what makes us fully human and identifies each of our individual human relationships and attachments as distinctive.

Uncomplicated grief encompasses a broad range of behaviors and feelings. Common grief reactions can include sadness, crying, anger, guilt and self-reproach, anxiety, loneliness, fatigue, problems with decision making, helplessness, shock, yearning, relief, numbness, physical reactions (stomach ache or lack of energy), disbelief, confusion, preoccupation, sleep disturbances, appetite disturbances, social withdrawal, or hyperactivity. Bereavement experts in the field suggest approximately 80% of those bereaved experience "uncomplicated grief" with an adaptive course of adjustment (Bonnano and Lilienfeld, 2008). Although there is no timeline for grief, most individuals begin to assimilate their loss and experience decreased grief reactions from 6 to 13 months after the death. The majority of survivors are able to integrate the loss into their lives and accommodate with resilience (Bonnano, 2004; Neimeyer, Burke, MacKay, and van Dyke Stringer, 2010). Conversely, 10% to 20% of bereaved persons suffer from complications which can prolong grief reactions, impair mental and physical health, and prohibit an adaptive course of healing (Shear, Frank, Houck, and Reynolds, 2005).

Military combat death presents many risk factors that lay an extremely strong foundation for complications in bereavement for survivors. Combat deaths can potentially lend themselves to a complicated grief process for survivors due to these factors:

- Sudden, violent death of the service member
- Death in a war zone or a foreign land, away from the family
- Delay in receiving information regarding circumstances of death
- Death notification
- Prolonged period of time between the death and the burial/interment
- Long periods of deployment separation prior to the death
- Condition of bodily remains, no remains, or multiple sets of remains
- Military burial rites and rituals
- Media involvement of the highly public deaths
- Young age of the deceased and young age of the survivors
- Paperwork and navigating bureaucracies
- Permanent decision making under extreme distress
- Multiple secondary losses bringing the possibility of the survivor experiencing "bereavement overload" (Kastenbaum, 1969): loss of housing or moving to a new school; loss of peers and social supports; involuntarily loss of military identity and community; potential loss of

income and employment; loss of family order; loss of practical support; loss of future potential, hopes, and dreams.

The literature suggests that those affected by sudden, violent deaths caused by accidents, suicide, homicide, acts of terrorism, and war are highly vulnerable to psychological trauma (Doka, 1996; Green, 2003) as well as the potential of developing complicated grief (Rando, 1996; Prigerson and Jacobs, 2001). The impact of bereavement with trauma can be long-lasting. Research suggests that violent death loss is found to predict symptoms of Posttraumatic Stress Disorder (PTSD), anxiety, depression, and health impairments which can further expose the survivor to a more enduring, distressed, and complicated bereavement. Most survivors expect to encounter grief, but they do not often understand that they are also suffering from symptoms of trauma. They feel as if they are "going crazy." Lu Redmond (1989), a prominent homicide researcher, observed that, "homicide survivors may present symptomatic behaviors characteristic of PTSD up to five years following a murdered loved one. This becomes a normal range of functioning for this distinct population" (p. 52).

Violent and traumatic deaths challenge a survivor's tasks of mourning by shaking his or her sense of self-efficacy, shattering the assumptive worldview, prohibiting expressions of anger and blame, and magnifying feelings of guilt (Worden, 2009). When trauma and grief overlap, unaddressed trauma impairs grief work and can interfere with the survivor's ability to understand and accept the reality of his or her family member's death, an essential first task in the ability to heal.

Traumatic death survivors can often feel "stuck" or "frozen in time." Sudden, untimely, or violent deaths produce circumstances in which posttraumatic stress responses take emotional priority in managing the overwhelming loss, horror, and profound sense of helplessness. Trying to cope with these post-trauma symptoms becomes the first priority, rather than working on normal expressions of grief, and the survivor's ability to grieve can be delayed.

Dealing with the dual effects of both grief and trauma can be an overwhelming experience for survivors who deal with, and alternate between, conflicting sets of thoughts, feelings, and reactions. It may take months or years for traumatic death survivors to truly begin to work on their grief.

While maintaining that grief is highly personal and each individual copes with loss in his or her own unique way, it is essential that anyone working with the bereaved, especially those who have suffered the combat death of a family service member, be aware of signs and symptoms of serious complications in bereavement, which can include:

- trouble accepting the loss;
- constant yearning or pining for the deceased years after the death;
- "feeling stuck" and not being able to move forward;
- inability to enjoy life;
- lack of trust;
- intrusive thoughts about the deceased;
- persistent inability to perform acts of daily functioning for months and years after the death;
- abuse of drugs and alcohol;
- symptoms of major depression and/or PTSD;
- medical neglect or failure to thrive;
- engagement in high-risk and self-destructive behaviors; and
- suicidal ideation and intent.

Warning signs and symptoms should be taken seriously and not be dismissed by the clinician as "just part of the grieving process," as they can be potentially life-threatening. Given the young age of this population, negative coping strategies may be more prevalent.

COMPLICATING MILITARY FACTORS THAT IMPACT SURVIVORS

> *The absence of next-of-kin notification, of graves registration procedures, of official provision for decent burial all seems unimaginable to us. The Civil War ended this neglect and established policies that led to today's commitment to identify and return every soldier killed in the line of duty (Faust, 2008, p. 271)*

The death of a family member in the U.S. military is fraught with complexities unlike those typically experienced in the civilian world (Carroll, 2001; Steen and Asaro, 2006), contributing to a potentially prolonged, distressing, and complicated grief process for many survivors. Combat death can bring additional challenges that families must face.

Acutely shocked and grief-stricken survivors—especially if they are the PNOK, SNOK and/or person authorized to direct disposition of remains (PADD)—are instantly confronted with the task of making difficult, permanent life decisions in the face of complex loss and trauma. They must navigate the intricate bureaucratic process involved with the dignified transfer of remains, disposition of the remains of a service member, and military burial rites and rituals. They must deal with personal effects of the deceased arriving from foreign lands, the public nature of the death (which sometimes includes protestors), and a substantial amount of paperwork associated with entitlements for survivor benefits, financial matters, and civilian wills and estates. These tasks often involve multiple civilian and larger macro systems of government, such as the DoD and VA.

Interpersonally, the survivor is coping with his or her own response to the service member's death while dealing with intrapersonal family dynamics. Family survivors often negotiate a roller coaster of emotions and complex factors within the context of multiple, intrapersonal familial, military, and organizational interactions.

The combat death of a loved one in the U.S. military leaves surviving family members with a coexisting series of crises as well as primary and secondary losses. The social changes that death may bring to the survivor may come very unexpectedly (Harrington-LaMorie, 2011). Factors surrounding a combat death in the present U.S. military that may compound the loss experience and predispose survivors to complications in their grief process will be elaborated next.

Death during deployment

One exceptional challenge faced by military families is that service members spend an extraordinary amount of time away from their families, both primary and extended, due to operational demands, predeployment trainings, and deployments. Military families become accustomed to their service member being gone for long periods of time. However, a combat deployment brings additional stress. The fear factor with combat death does not start with the notification of the death of the service member, but starts with the actual deployment. Along with additional strains related to a combat deployment, there is the constant worry by family members about injury or death. Combat deaths can occur days, weeks, or months into a deployment and, for some, near the very end.

Parents of service members often report having increased levels of fear due to their geographic and legal disconnection from the military unit in which their children serve. If the service member is married, communication about what is occurring with that service member is heavily dependent on communication with the spouse of the service member, who has the support of Family Readiness Officers (FROs) and other military families. The quality of this relationship can serve reciprocally, as one of support or additional stress.

Surviving spouses and children may rely on the military community as their primary support system, as most live far away from their families of origin (with the exception of most National Guard and Reserves). Since the service member was most likely far away from their parents, siblings, family and friends for extended periods of time prior to the death, last words and moments spent together may have been few and far between.

Deploying service members who have children sometimes unwittingly place the responsibility of care on their oldest child by saying things such as, "Take care of your mom and siblings while I am gone." When a death occurs, this last request may be perceived to remain in effect forever by the child and prohibit them from ever "acting like a kid" again for fear of betraying that promise to a deceased parent (Beard, 2008).

The experience of multiple previous separations makes it harder for family members to realize or acknowledge that their loved one is gone forever when they die during a combat deployment. Otherwise known as "deployment-delayed" grief, survivors can employ high levels of defense mechanisms to cope and create a subconscious denial that their service member has died, instead telling themselves that they are still "away" on deployment. The reality often hits the survivor with acute grief reactions (even after a memorial or burial has taken place) when the unit returns and the service member is not with them. This delay in grief can often interfere with normative grieving processes for survivors (Steen and Asaro, 2006).

The fact that service members die fighting in foreign lands and outside the presence of their families contributes to a survivor's vulnerability to experiencing feelings of ambiguous loss. Ambiguous loss creates a complicated grief by making the ability to accept the reality of the loss extremely difficult for survivors who are unable to physically see or identify that their family member has died (Boss, 2010). This situation may be alleviated if bodily remains are found and returned home.

Circumstances of death and condition of bodily remains

The manner in which someone dies can have a deeply profound and enduring impact on survivors. Family survivors of service members who have been killed in action report a full range of feelings and emotions centered on the circumstance of their service member's death. While some find meaning in death in service, many report experiencing the same grief reactions and long-term challenges of those who have experienced a family member dying by homicide. The human-to-human element of the death cannot be discounted in the survivor's grieving process because it happened within the context of a war. Bereavement following death by sudden or violent means brings a psychological and emotional impact to the survivor that is a synergistic experience of both grief and trauma (Neria and Litz, 2004).

Combat deaths are overwhelmingly violent and involve multiple causes that can bring minimal or massive trauma to the body. Bodily remains could be intact, fragmented, retrieved bit by bit, never found, or deemed as not viewable. If not found or not viewable, this can further complicate the survivor's grief, as the survivor can deny or delay the reality of the death. Boss (2006), who did groundbreaking work with family members of union workers lost in the terrorist attacks of 9/11, makes the connection between ambiguous loss and trauma. Recent research suggests that there may be benefits to being allowed to view a loved one's body after a sudden death (Chapple and Ziebland, 2010). The ability for survivors to get up close to the deceased affords them the opportunity to orient themselves to the reality of the death and acknowledge the loss. This is the essential first task in Worden's (2009) tasks of mourning.

The decision to allow authorized family members to view bodily remains is given to a family member, and it is a decision solely based on their own judgment about what they believe they can tolerate. For some family members, seeing the only remaining foot and ankle of their service member brought them to a place, emotionally and psychologically, where they could begin a healing process. For others, it caused them further harm. It is a highly subjective choice.

Clearly, the circumstances of a service member's death and the condition of the bodily remains have long-term impacts on a survivor's grief and bereavement experience.

Death notification

The U.S. military formally notifies the PNOK and SNOK that their service member has died. However, if the death is highly public, with media coverage, survivors may unofficially know prior to the official notification team. The military notification team usually arrives in an official government vehicle, wearing cleaned and decorated uniforms. Typically, they come in pairs, a notification officer and a chaplain.

Death notification brings a message and a messenger that changes a survivor's life forever—the experience of the loss of an assumptive world which alters a person's life and state of being. The world they once knew is forever changed. Receiving and delivering this news is painful and difficult for both the survivor and notification team. Even with the best training and sensitivity, notifying a family that a service member has suddenly died can be a "primary" traumatic event. The shock of the news can overwhelm the internal resources of the survivor, triggering a variety of individual responses. Shutting down, screaming, acting numb, crying hysterically, or behaving with intense rage can all be responses to hearing the news.

For mental health practitioners, the way survivors recall the event can be as varied as the emotional reactions; they can remember nothing, vague details, or with pinpointed accuracy every detail of the moment. Retelling the story of the death notification can create a reactivation response for survivors; it is important that both caregivers and survivors are aware of this posttraumatic response. Letting survivors tell the story at their own pace, and preparing for unexpected grief reactions and validating distressing emotions, even years after the death, are important. Death notification begins the long-term impact of a combat death.

The Casualty Officer

After notification of their service member's death, it is the Casualty Assistance Officer (CAO) or Casualty Assistance Call Officer (CACO) that often becomes the PNOK's main source of comfort and support.

It is the casualty officer who arranges the family's visit to Dover Air Force Base in Dover, DE (if the family so desires) to witness the return of their family service member to the United States and dignified transfer of remains. Seeing the flag-draped coffin is often the family's first opportunity to visually and emotionally acknowledge their service member's death.

The casualty officer assists the family in negotiating the multiple events that occur in a relatively quick succession following their return home from Dover. The casualty officer's primary roles are to meet the immediate needs of the next of kin; assist with return, transfer, and burial of remains; assist with handling the media; navigate the bureaucratic process; assist with paperwork; process benefit claims; and assist with applying for requests for investigation reports. The CAO/CACO's commitment in working with the surviving family members varies in time from three months to a year. Once the paperwork is submitted and the last benefit is claimed, the job of the casualty officer is over.

A secondary loss can occur when the casualty officer separates from the family. If a close relationship between the family and the casualty officer develops, families can experience further distress if the casualty officer's next orders are a deployment to a combat area. Long-term case work for families may still be required once the casualty officer is relieved of duty. Programs such as the Tragedy Assistance Program for Survivors (TAPS) and the Army Survivor Outreach Services Program (SOS) provide such care.

Funerals, memorials, and burials

The family is notified within 24 hours of a casualty; however, with casualties from Iraq and Afghanistan, it may take some time before remains are identified and sent home. It can take military families two to three months (and sometimes longer) to bury or have a funeral service for their service member. These prolonged periods may be attributed to factors such as long waiting periods for national cemeteries, transfer of bodies, condition or location of remains, decisions on group burials, and medical investigations. It is not atypical for families to wait for several months for burial service while these complicating practical details are being sorted. Families will often have a memorial service before making any decisions about funeral arrangements with their casualty officer.

There are many rites and rituals associated with a military funeral in a military cemetery. The structure provided by the military may seem distant and cold to some surviving family members, but can provide comfort in a time of shock and trauma for others. Killed-in-action combat deaths have explicit acknowledgments and honors by the military and are held in the highest regard. Being the family survivor of a service member who dies in combat can bring with it much support, but also many burdens.

Given the high profile of deaths from Iraq and Afghanistan, families are invited to attend multiple memorials, services, and national holiday events throughout the years after a loved one's death. In addition, some military units tape memorial services and send them to the family. Because of the number of events and the expectations of those in attendance to encapsulate a permanent vision of a grief-stricken survivor, military families can tend to become "professional grievers."

Immediate impact to survivors

The practical and emotional demands on the individual survivor and family who are suddenly notified of a service member's combat death are extraordinary. From the moment of death notification, the complex decisions regarding the death begin.

As noted earlier, designated family members of the fallen are invited to attend the dignified transfer of remains at Dover AFB. In many cases, the family must decide quickly if they want to attend the transfer, as well as whether or not to allow media to film.

As with any death, notifying other family members is a struggle for the surviving PNOK. The suddenness of the death often robs the survivor of the opportunity to get real-time professional or trusted help for a critical need. The violence of the death often leaves families questioning what and how much to tell without causing any undue further harm. When young children are among the family members to be notified, some parents may delay relating detailed information to their children and may need assistance in the next few days, weeks, months or years after the death. Grief counselors and therapists have been valuable in assisting families with this process. Local hospices and grief centers can be helpful resources, as well as national organizations such as The Dougy Center, The National Child Traumatic Stress Network, and TAPS.

Immediate complex life-altering decisions need to be made within hours, days, and short weeks following a service member's death, an event which was already sudden and vastly unanticipated. Experts in grief suggest that survivors should not make any life-altering decisions within the first six months after the death of a loved one or significant relationship (Creagan, 2012). The military is beginning to recognize this best practice suggestion, but sometimes surviving spouses are faced with decisions on moving, monetary benefits, handling personal effects and household goods, and schooling for children, all within the first three to twelve months after a service member has died, depending upon where they are stationed. If a death happens on a foreign post or base, dependent survivors may need to make these decisions within 90 days.

Media attention and political protestors

Combat deaths are highly publicized in the media. The media can be a very unwelcome or welcome part of a survivor's journey. "Faces of the Fallen" are often put on public display in the news and social media, and their lives and their family's stories become narratives for public consumption. Family members often speak of receiving condolence cards from the public, which for some seems caring, and for others is uncomfortable.

Because of the public nature of combat deaths and political nature of the wars, some families are subjected to vindictive protests at their service member's funeral and internment. The grieving family members are forced to endure this behavior at a time when they are least able to cope with additional distress (Beard, 2008). Groups such as the Patriot Guard can be available to assist families at funerals to block the sight of protestors.

Age of descendents/age of survivors

The majority of service members killed in Iraq and Afghanistan are enlisted men under the age of 30. As discussed earlier, they are survived by young parents, young families, and young siblings. Like wars throughout history, young widowhood has been an indelible mark of these current wars. Images of young mothers surrounded by now fatherless children are no different from those images captured from the Civil War. Letters from bereaved mothers who speak of the untimely loss of their sons and daughters resonate today as they have with every generation of war mothers.

The unexpected, tragic, and untimely death of a young adult places the survivor in a position that is out-of-sync with their developmental phase. With the average life expectancy of Americans being 77 years old (CDC, 2009), young adult loss presents unique challenges to surviving families. Various factors contributing to this include a lack of similar others who have experienced the same type of loss; this is especially true for families who have had loved ones killed in combat. Given that .0017% of American service members have been killed in combat during the wars in Iraq and Afghanistan, the surviving community is a rare, unique subpopulation in American society (DMDC, 2012; U.S. Census Bureau, 2012). Other factors include an inexperience with previous deaths, especially that of a spouse or child at a young age, and a limited and geographically dispersed peer group. Because of these limitations, young adults coping with loss may not have mentors or role models to provide social support and model coping skills (Walter and McCoyd, 2009).

Distinctive problems plague families who experience the loss of a young adult. For those who suffered the combat death of a family service member, some of these difficulties can include future losses, changed roles, challenges with identity, financial issues, and changed family order. Surviving spouses experience additional challenges: raising children as an "only parent," loss of a male role model for young children, the potential loss of never being able to have children, and the possible question of remarriage before the age of 57, which can negatively affect benefits and entitlements.

When a young adult dies, family roles change, identity within the family may change, and familial developmental tasks are challenged as they grieve the death of this person throughout their life (Walter and McCoyd, 2009). Grieving someone who dies an untimely death has an inherent challenge in bereavement which places the survivor in the position of a prolonged journey of grieving multiple losses across the lifespan.

When a service member is killed in combat as an adolescent or young adult, the immediate impacts involve grieving the past and the present with that person. The long-term impact of a young, untimely death is being confronted with grieving their future, especially during developmental milestones. For many surviving parents, a wedding of their friend's child can trigger grief, sadness and thoughts that "this should have been my son at 30." They may also fear for the safety and mortality of their surviving children or grieve the loss of an only child. For surviving spouses, the waves of grief may come at the high school graduations of their children or wedding anniversary dates. Dating relationships can become difficult if the new person in the relationship feels threatened "filling the shoes" of a war hero. For surviving siblings, grief often comes in the form of holidays, where a table of six is now set for a table of five. Surviving siblings must also contend with living in the shadow of a sibling war hero, which can be a source of conflicting feelings of both pride and jealousy. For surviving children, there are constant loss reminders associated with all the events that mom or dad should be attending with them, such as baseball games, recitals, graduations, school dances, and their own weddings. Untimely deaths end the life of the deceased early, yet can prolong the journey for survivors over their lifetime.

Commitment to service

The survivor's viewpoint of the service member's military career is an essential determining factor, so a service member's commitment to service must be explored with each survivor, as it can be a potential risk or healing factor as each person grieves. Some may be angry at their loved one's choice to enlist, especially during a time of war. Survivors may also feel abandoned and cheated if their service member chose to re-enlist. Pride in service can be a healing factor, but can also be confusing because of the dichotomy between the devastating negative emotions of grief and immense pride in their family member's service. For some, there is additional anger directed at the military that sent their family member to war or the enemy who killed them. Some survivors find it uncomfortable to speak of the pride of service outside the military context, because many civilians can't identify with it or mistake it for a lack of sorrow.

After the flag is folded

A significant ritual at a military funeral is when the American flag draping the coffin is carefully folded and handed to the family. When the flag is finally folded and the service member is laid to rest, support for the family diminishes and life moves forward. The survivor is now faced with the reality of the impact of their service member's death, often many weeks or months after the actual death has occurred.

The combat death of a family service member subjects surviving family members to a series of losses associated with the death. In addition to the actual death, losses include a loss of their way of life and identity associated with this life, loss of their housing (if on base or post), and loss of their greater military community. Surviving spouses and children may feel a sense of disjointedness as they are given an immediate "involuntary" discharge by the military, while remaining tied to the military by benefits and entitlements. Surviving parents and siblings living in the civilian community may have a sense of profound isolation from a community that understands. These sudden, multiple, and compounding losses may bring with them a profound sense of loneliness and disenfranchisement for the surviving family. National holidays that memorialize deceased service members and veterans can be helpful or a continued trigger of pain. Since family survivors also represent the service member hero, they may be asked on multiple occasions to attend events in their honor. Given the young age of service members killed in combat and their survivors, this can continue for decades.

Disenfranchised grief and the military

Doka's (1988) work in disenfranchised grief can also be applied to families of those who are killed in combat. A survivor's grief can often be disenfranchised by society, met with the nonchalant attitude that their loved one chose to join the military, especially during a time of war, and their death should be considered "anticipated." Statements such as, "What did you expect? He joined the infantry during a time of war," are the type of responses often encountered by family survivors. Survivors are somehow expected to be prepared to anticipate death with this high-risk job. However, the impact of the loss is no less powerful or significant to the individuals who have survived the deceased.

CLINICAL ISSUES

First and foremost, do no harm. If you are a clinician or care provider who has not worked with survivors of sudden or violent death, this should not be your first case. Survivor cases can be complicated, graphic in nature, and involve an intense amount of complex grief and trauma. As a reminder, if the survivor's presenting problems are beyond one's skill set, refer, refer, and refer. Referrals to grief therapists can be found by contacting a local hospice or Vet Center, or through the Association for Death Education and Counseling.

It is important for general practitioners in community-based care to check in with themselves about their own feelings concerning military service and the war, and how this may or may not create issues within the context of a therapeutic or clinical relationship. Identifying, recognizing, and managing countertransference is essential to the therapeutic alliance and relationship.

A key factor in working with anyone in the midst of grief, loss, and transition is being mindful of the cultural factors of their population. There is a unique culture to the military and an even more distinctive culture to the survivor population and combat-death subpopulation. The culturally competent practitioner should become as informed as possible and show a willingness to learn from the survivor about their experiences and cultural influences.

Certain survivors find a continued connection to the military and veterans organizations helpful and healing. Some volunteer their experience and stories in trainings to schools, organizations, and even the military community.

On the other hand, some survivors want nothing to do with the military or veterans organizations. If desired, a practitioner can help encourage healthy connections and boundaries with the military and veteran community. Many survivors create foundations and organizations in honor of their service member, which helps make meaning of the death, find an enduring connection with the deceased, and engage in living and moving forward. These activities can be helpful, but should always be considered with caution so that survivors are not distracting themselves with activity and prohibiting the work that grief requires.

Psycho-education is also an important part of the process. Books and magazines on personal accounts and peer support from survivors of combat death can be helpful. Professional books on grief, sudden loss, violent death, trauma, mass casualties, and those based on loss of relationship type (e.g., death of a spouse, child, sibling) can also be of assistance to survivors in their healing.

Self-help and support groups can be helpful. However, practitioners should be mindful to refer survivors to groups in which members are similar in age and circumstance of death (violent or sudden death). Most survivors report feeling disconnected from civilian support groups, where a military death is unique, and they find difficulty finding reciprocity of support or an inherent understanding with another survivor. When military survivors do attend support groups, it is commonly reported that they feel the most similarities with survivors of homicide deaths.

Interventional strategies and suggested resources

Interventional strategies in working with bereaved military families include individual therapy, peer support, support groups, cognitive behavioral therapy, prescription medication (under the direction of a physician), Eye Movement Desensitization and Reprocessing (EMDR), evidence-based trauma therapies, complicated grief therapy, and suicide assessment. Complementary modalities of care include art therapy, sleep review/sleep therapy, breathing techniques, meditation, guided imagery, massage, nutritional support, and exercise.

If a survivor is a parent, spouse, sibling, or child of a U.S. Armed Services member, Reservist, or National Guardsman who was killed in action, he or she is eligible for bereavement counseling through the Department of Veterans Affairs Vet Centers (www.vetcenter.va.gov). Long-term support for surviving Army families can be obtained through Army Survivor Outreach Service, under Family Programs and Services (http://www.myarmyonesource.com).

The power of peer support is an underutilized but highly recognized area of healing and support for surviving military families. TAPS, which was founded in 1994 by a military widow, provides peer-based programs for adults and children and is a considerable source of care for the family, regardless of the circumstance of the death and relationship to the deceased. Congressionally chartered advocacy groups, such as American Gold Star Mothers, Inc. and Gold Star Wives of America, Inc., along with the post 9/11 American Widow Project, all provide a peer network for families of a service member killed in combat.

Jill Harrington-LaMorie, DSW, LCSW is currently the Senior Field Researcher on a Congressionally Directed Medical Research Project, "The Impact of a Service Member's Death: A National Study of Bereavement in Military Families," being conducted at Uniformed Services University of the Health Services Center for the Study of Traumatic Stress, Bethesda, MD. Dr. Harrington-LaMorie is the former Director of Professional Education at the Tragedy Assistance Program for Survivors (TAPS). Dr. Harrington-LaMorie is one of the first published authors on the subject of bereavement in U.S. military families. She is a member of The National Association of Social Workers and serves on the National Board of the Association for Death Education and Counseling.

Betsy Beard is a multi-award-winning author. Her writing career began on October 14, 2004, following the notification that her only son had been killed in action in Iraq. Shortly thereafter she discovered Tragedy Assistance Program for Survivors (TAPS). She began contributing articles about survivorship to TAPS Magazine, *as well as to* Living with Loss Magazine, *and Hospice Foundation of America's* Living with Grief *program. In 2008, Ms. Beard became the editor for* TAPS Magazine. *Ms. Beard is the author of* Klinger, A Story of Honor and Hope, *the Military Writers Society of America's 2011 Gold Medal winner for Children's Books.*

For their invaluable contributions of background and anecdotal information, the authors wish to thank:

Betsy Coffin, *Surviving Spouse*, 1st Sgt. Christopher D. Coffin, U.S. Army, 1st Battalion, 64th Armor Regiment, 2nd Brigade Combat Team, 3rd Infantry Division, Fort Stewart, GA, killed 7/1/2003, Baghdad, Iraq; **Maggie McCloud**, *Surviving Spouse*, Lt. Colonel Joseph Trane McCloud, U.S. Marine Corps, 2nd Battalion, 3rd Marine Regiment, 3rd Marine Division, III Marine Expeditionary Force, Kaneohe Bay, HI, killed 12/3/2006, Lake Qadisiyah, Iraq; **Donna Engeman**, *Surviving Spouse*, Chief Warrant Officer, U.S. Army, 1st Battalion, 312th Regiment, 30th Enhanced Separate Brigade, Clinton, NC, killed 5/18/2006, Baghdad, Iraq; **Meredith McMackin**, *Surviving Mother*, Corporal Julian M. Woodall, U.S. Marine Corps, 3rd Battalion, 10th Marine Regiment, 2nd Marine Division, II Marine Expeditionary Force, Camp LeJeune, NC, killed 5/22/2007, Zanti, Iraq; **Myra Rintamaki**, *Surviving Mother*, Corporal Steven A. Rintamaki, 3rd Battalion, 1st Marine Regiment, 1st Marine Division, 1 Marine Expeditionary Force, killed 9/16/2004, Al Anbar Province, Iraq.

This chapter is dedicated to all military surviving families; those who tend to the care of survivors and those who tend to the care of the deceased; the countless number of fellow service members whose grief for their comrades goes unrecognized; and to all those who have died in military service to America.

REFERENCES

Antonov-Ovseyenko, A. (1981). *The time of Stalin: Portrait of a tyranny*. New York, NY: Harper & Row.

Beard, B. (2008). Military Children and Grief. In K.J. Doka & A.S. Tucci (Eds.), *Living with Grief: Children and Adolescents*. Washington, DC: Hospice Foundation of America.

Bonanno, G.A. (2004). Loss, trauma, and human resilience: Have we underestimated the human capacity to thrive after extremely aversive events? *American Psychologist, 59*(1), 20–28.

Bonnano, G.A., & Lilienfeld, S.O. (2008). When grief counseling is effective and when it's not. *Professional Psychology: Research & Practice, 39*(3), 377-378.

Boss, P. (2006). *Loss, trauma and resilience: Therapeutic work with ambiguous loss*. New York: NY: W.W. Norton & Company.

Boss, P. (2010). The trauma and complicated grief of ambiguous loss. *Pastoral Psychology 50*(2), 137-145.

Carroll, B. (2001). How the military family copes with a death. In O.D. Weeks & C. Johnson (Eds.), *When all the friends have gone: A guide for aftercare providers* (pp. 173-183). Amityville, NY: Baywood.

Chapple, A., & Ziebland, S. (2010). Viewing the body after bereavement due to a traumatic death: Qualitative study in the UK. *British Medical Journal, 340*, c2032.

Creagan, E.T. (2012). *Grief: A Mayo Clinic doctor confronts painful emotions*. Mayo Clinic Online. Retrieved October 31, 2012 from http://www.mayoclinic.com/health/grief/HQ00771

Defense Manpower Data Center (2012). Military casualty information Retrieved October 31, 2012 from http://siadapp.dmdc.osd.mil/personnel/CASUALTY/castop.htm

Doka, K. (Ed.). (1996). *Living with grief after sudden loss: Suicide, homicide, accident, heart attack, stroke*. New York, NY: Routledge (Taylor & Francis Group).

Doka, K. (Ed.). (1998). *Disenfranchised grief: Recognizing hidden sorrow*. Lexington, MA: Lexington Books.

Faust, D.G. (2008). *This republic of suffering: Death and the American Civil War*. New York, NY: Random House, Inc.

Green, B.L. (2003). *Trauma interventions in war and peace: Prevention, practice and policy*. New York, NY: Kluwer Academic/Plenum Publishing.

Harrington-LaMorie, J. (2011). Operation Iraqi Freedom/Operation Enduring Freedom: Exploring Wartime Death & Bereavement. *Social Work in Health Care, 50*, 543-563.

Harrington-LaMorie, J. & McDevitt-Murphy, M. (2011). Traumatic death in the United States military: Initiating the dialogue on war-related loss. In R.A. Neimeyer, H. Winokuer, D. Harris, & G. Thornton (Eds.), *Grief and bereavement in contemporary society: Bridging research and practice*. New York, NY: Routledge.

Kastenbaum, R.J. (1969). Death and bereavement in later life. In A.H. Kutscher (Ed.), *Death and bereavement* (pp. 27-54). Springfield, IL: Thomas.

Neimeyer, R.A., Burke, L.A., Mackay, M.M., & van Dyke Stringer, J.G. (2010). Grief therapy and the reconstruction of meaning: From principles to practice. *Journal of Contemporary Psychotherapy, 40*(2), 73–83.

Neria, Y., & Litz, B.T. (2004). Bereavement by traumatic means: The complex synergy of trauma and grief. *Journal of Loss and Trauma, 9*, 73–87.

Prigerson, H.G., & Jacobs, S. (2001). Traumatic grief as a distinct disorder. In M.S. Stroebe, R.O. Hansson, W. Stroebe, & H. Schut (Eds.), *Handbook of bereavement research: Consequences, coping and care* (pp. 613–645). Washington, DC: American Psychological Association.

Rando, T.A. (1993). *Treatment of Complicated Mourning*. Champaign, IL: Research Press.

Redmond, L.M. (1989). *Surviving: When someone you love was murdered—A professional's guide to group grief therapy for families and friends of murder victims*. Clearwater, FL: Psychological Consultation and Education Services.

Shear, K., Frank, E., Houck, P.R., & Reynolds, C.F. (2005). Treatment of complicated grief: A randomized controlled trial. *Journal of the American Medical Association, 293*(21), 2601–2608.

Steen, J.M., & Asaro, M.R. (2006). *Military widow: A survival guide*. Annapolis, MD: Naval Institute Press.

U.S. Census Bureau (2012). U.S population. Retrieved October 31, 2012 from http://quickfacts.census.gov/qfd/states/00000.html

Walter, C.A., & McCoyd, J.L.M. (2009). *Grief and loss across the lifespan: A biopsychosocial perspective*. New York, NY: Springer Publishing Company.

Worden, J.W. (2009). *Grief counseling and grief therapy: A handbook for the mental health practitioner* (4th Edition). New York, NY: Springer Publishing Co.

Zinner, E.S., & Williams, M.B. (Eds.). (1999). *When a community weeps: Case studies in group survivorship*. Philadelphia, PA: Brunner/Mazel (Taylor & Francis Group).

Author's Note: Since the assessment and treatment of complicated and traumatic bereavement is a rapidly growing and emerging field, it is recommended that readers explore the work of experts such as M. Katherine Shear, MD; Edward K. Rynearson, MD; Robert Neimeyer, PhD, and Holly S. Prigerson; Charles Figley, PhD; and Ilona Pivar, PhD, for further information.

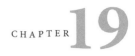

Voices
A Military Widow

Joanne Steen

I am a military widow. It is not an identity I sought, nor a lifestyle I chose.

I remember when I had it all: a new marriage glistening in its honeymoon aura, a dream job that was the highlight of my career, and a new home with a sunny bedroom begging for a crib and a rocking chair. Life was better than good, or so I thought. My happy life exploded—just like the helicopter my husband was flying—on an innocent Friday afternoon leading into a much-anticipated Father's Day weekend.

My husband, Navy Lieutenant Ken Steen, his co-pilot, and their five-man air crew, were coming home from a training mission when the helicopter Ken was flying exploded in midair, according to a slew of eyewitnesses. All seven souls on board the aircraft perished.

Denial and disbelief ruled the remnants of my once innocent Friday, and the first inklings of reality invaded the night. Ken and his crew were breaking news. Unwilling to sleep, I sat glued to the TV, where CNN showed salvage crews removing bodies and pieces of wreckage that was the aircraft my husband flew just a few hours earlier. Daylight brought the morning newspaper with its screaming headlines: NAVY COPTER EXPLODES: 7 DIE. And there was Ken's picture below the headline, with his trademark smile and sparkling eyes, looking very much alive and not very dead. Shock replaced denial. I couldn't deal with this overdose of reality.

I was no stranger to death. I came from a large family where a relative or two would arrive or depart in any given year, just like celestial clockwork. However, nothing in my life—not even my own father's death six weeks earlier—could have prepared me for the sudden, traumatic, and public death of my young military husband. A military death is complex, complicated, and just plain messy. I learned this lesson in real time.

I buried Ken with full military honors in a veterans cemetery established by President Abraham Lincoln to bury the Civil War dead. Ken's funeral was the first of seven that week. The military honors—the playing of *Taps*, the twenty-one gun salute, the folded flag off my husband's coffin, the missing man flyby—all were fitting tributes to a service member who was killed in the line of duty. But the tribute I held closest to my heart was a personal one. At the cemetery, as the squadron filed past Ken's coffin for the last time, each pilot removed his coveted "Wings of Gold" and placed his Navy wings on Ken's coffin—the ultimate tribute to one of their own. Actions speak volumes. Mere words could never convey the depth of their respect. Or the depth of their loss.

I foolishly thought that once the funeral and squadron memorial were behind me, the worst was over. I was so naive. Ken's crash was my ticket into a world of living hell. A hell, I was to learn, with no boundaries and no escape. I remember a well-intentioned squadron girlfriend telling me at Ken's funeral I should now "get on with my life." At the time, I didn't understand that her clichéd comment was for her benefit, not mine. How was I supposed to "get on with my life" when I just buried the heart and soul of my future? Incomprehensible devastation replaced the love and the life I had known and cherished just a day or two earlier. That sunny bedroom—the one with high hopes of becoming a nursery—became the repository for death's paperwork: autopsy reports, accident investigations, innumerable forms, sympathy cards and the crisply folded flag I cradled at my young husband's graveside.

A military death comes with its own baggage. It is usually unexpected, potentially traumatic, possibly in another country or away from the duty station, complicated by marriage, publicized in the media, compounded by the military bureaucracy, and enveloped in commitment to duty and country. Our service members are young, well-trained, and in good health. They think they're invincible, and, as family members, we think so, too. They are a part of something bigger than themselves, a greater purpose, for they have sworn to protect and defend America from all its enemies, foreign and domestic. They often die in violent ways, leaving behind unrecognizable remains. They die in distant places and foreign countries, denying surviving family members the opportunity to go find the exact spot where their loved one died and "see for themselves."

By military survivor standards, I was one of the "lucky" widows, depending on how one defines luck. Not only was I able to sneak a peek at my husband's remains, but I also could visit the crash site, which was just a few miles from our home. This was a blessing and a curse. On one hand, I had real, visible proof that this devastating news, initially delivered by a casualty officer, was true. I went to the crash site as soon as the military allowed me. It was, and always will be, sacred ground to me, because it owns the final moments of my young husband's life. In an odd sort of way I felt peacefully connected to it, and I guess I always will. On the other hand, having the crash site as my almost next-door neighbor kept the image of an exploding helicopter in my psyche for a very long time. It took years of focus to replace that image with one rooted in the present.

Military loss leaves a wounded body, mind, and spirit in its survivors, with lots of jagged edges exposed to the elements of American life. A survivor cannot look at America the same way. While it's the service member who makes the ultimate sacrifice, it's the surviving family member who bears the burden of living that sacrifice, in big and small ways, each and every day. Military traditions and symbols of America, embedded into the collective American unconscious, now aggravate those jagged edges of loss in ways never imagined by the non-survivor community. *The Star Spangled Banner*, sung at innumerable professional and recreational events, becomes a personal reminder of a survivor's military loss and can ignite a significant emotional event, as easily as the 30-second snippets of a military homecoming, or a military funeral, on the evening news. Uniformed military personnel, perhaps unseen or unnoticed before, now pop up everywhere, just like hardy summer dandelions. Each one is a slap-in-the-face reminder that your service member is dead. Because of the significance of military service, our nation has not one, but two, federal holidays to honor America's living and dead veterans, Memorial Day and Veterans Day. These days are revered by families of the fallen, because America publically acknowledges and appreciates the sacrifices of our veterans. For surviving military families though, every day is a Memorial Day.

I wasn't prepared for the long list of secondary losses that accompanied my loss of Ken, nor for the power these secondary losses yielded. In addition to the obvious ones, such as the loss of our planned family, the predictability of life and my sense of safety, I lost much more. Just a few days after the crash—and long before I bought into the realization that this nightmare was true—I was escorted to the personnel office on the Navy base to surrender my military ID card that identified me as Ken's spouse. It was replaced by another military ID with my new identity: URW, which in military speak translates to Un-Remarried Widow. My identity as Ken's wife had been officially taken away from me, long before I was ready to give up being known as his wife.

I also lost my military way of life. While the squadron rallied around the crash families, there came a time when they needed to refocus on the business of living. There were missions to fly, replacement pilots to train, and babies to raise. Without Ken, I was no longer a part of this squadron, and the other squadron wives and I drifted apart. After all, I was a powerful reminder that good men die young and fate was not fickle. Like most military widows, I was suspended between two worlds—there's no good place for widows within the active-duty military lifestyle, and my former civilian life seemed like an alien culture.

I don't know what motivated me forward in the dark years after the crash. But whatever it was, I'm grateful for it. Peace of mind came in fleeting moments, little wisps of comfort that darted hither and yon through my psyche. I recall asking a veteran military widow how I would know I was getting better and she said simply, "When you get up one morning and Ken isn't the first person you think about." It happened one morning, without drama or fanfare.

A few years after the crash, the Navy approached me about plans to erect a memorial helicopter to the fated crew of NW601, the crash helicopter, on the Navy base where Ken and the rest of the guys had been stationed. I was delighted, for it meant Ken and the crew would not simply fade away into the nameless void of casualty statistics. On the fifth anniversary of the crash, the Navy and I dedicated an exact replica of the crash helicopter to the NW601 crew. In my dedication speech, I told the audience:

> I know what one of the crew members would say, if he were standing here—in my shoes—today. He would tell us to remember him as he lived, not as he died. He would say to live and love again with a renewed appreciation for this gift of life…
> I know the greatest tribute we could pay to the crew of NW601 would be to live our lives to the fullest.

The road from military wife to military widow to a woman of my own right was the toughest challenge I've ever faced. I didn't do it perfectly; some days I wondered if I could do it at all. But I made it, just like all those brave military widows before me. I changed careers, fell in and out of love a couple of times, and tried to remain optimistic about life.

I'm happy today. I won't use the worn-out cliché and label it a new chapter or even a new life. It's the same life I've always had, just shaped by the joys and tragedies that occur in everyone's life. I've found the second great love of my life, and discovered it's never too late to live happily ever after. It's a different love, one that was robbed of innocence and baptized by jet fuel and blood, a long time ago.

I believe I'll meet Ken again one day. When I do, I hope and pray he'll give me a big hug and tell me he's proud of the way I faced the future and pressed on without him.

Joanne Steen, MS, NCC, is an author, instructor, and speaker on line-of-duty loss with Grief Solutions, LLC. She is the award-winning co-author of Military Widow: A Survival Guide *(Naval Institute Press, 2006) and the author of the forthcoming* Military Parents: We Regret to Inform You. *She welcomes your comments at JMSteen@griefsolutions.net.*

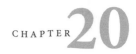

CHAPTER 20

Military Suicide: Counseling Survivors

Antoon A. Leenaars

D estruction and violence are inherent in war. An often-used legacy on war stress is of the 19th-century Prussian general and war theorist, Carl Gottfried von Clausewitz. The general described and used the word "friction" to name the stresses of combat. War stress is unforgiving. Suicide is an all too frequent response (Leenaars, 2013). This was true after the American Civil War, and not since that U.S. war have we seen so many of our heroes die by their own hand. One U.S. military personnel has died by suicide every day so far in 2012 (Thompson, 2012). This is an epidemic that must be addressed.

System, Culture, and the Military

Who is the soldier? What is at the core of the unique military system? The armed forces system/culture has its own characteristics, patterns, and associations. Probably one of the most obvious facts is that being a soldier is an identity, a self. On the identity of the warrior, Hall (2011) writes:

> On a deeper, perhaps more psychological level, many who join the military feel a need to "merge their identity with that of the warrior"....so it is not uncommon for young men to merge their identity with that of a warrior by being a part of something meaningful, which is a motivation to join the military. (p. 34)

There are greater commonalities than differences in suicide around the world (Leenaars, 2007). However, there are also critical differences. In collective cultures, such as the military, there are a great deal more indirect expressions, unconscious processes, dissembling, and masking. The collective culture encourages warriors, and thus suicidal soldiers and veterans, to adhere to core values and moral tradition, including in matters of death and suicide.

There can be great stigmatization, even with some believing that the suicidal soldier or veteran is not a true warrior.

People in the military take pride in their collective system, but maybe for suicidal soldiers, it fosters not communicating the intent, not even being conscious of individual pain, and not seeking help. The suicidal state is, therefore, more veiled, clouded, or guarded. This is called dissembling or masking and is a significant factor in suicide risk in the military (Leenaars, 2013). Military training has been seen as indoctrination. Recruits begin on the very first day "to more actively integrate the values of the group into their own individual worldviews" (Christian, Stivers, and Sammons, 2009, p. 42). The dehumanization created by these processes facilitates the ability to kill, sometimes beyond the context of combat. Violence is acceptable. Is it only in battle? Can it be towards oneself, in honor? Is military suicide altruistic?

This indoctrination does not result in only negative consequences. It creates resilience or hardiness, and hardiness is known to mediate the relationship between combat exposure and stress, Posttraumatic Stress Disorder (PTSD), depression, and suicide risk. It allows one to persevere, despite the war friction.

SUICIDE AND A SYSTEM MODEL

It is estimated that 1.6 million people die by violence each year. Almost half (800,000) of these are suicides; one-third are homicides (530,000); and one-fifth (320,000) are war-related (WHO, 2002). No single factor or event explains why so many people are violent. Violence is multidetermined and complex. Suicide, homicide, and war-related deaths are not like water, where all water freezes at 32 degrees Fahrenheit. Suicide, war-related deaths, etc., are the result of interplay of individual, relationship, social, cultural, and environmental factors. This is sometimes called *the ecological model*. The model has been applied to a vast array of behaviors, most recently violence, including self-directed violence; for example, suicide (WHO, 2002). The model simply suggests that there are different levels, i.e., individual, relationship, community, and societal, that influence war-related violence, deaths, and suicide, and fortunately, by implication, one can understand and address violence at various levels.

Suicide is self-directed lethal violence and a multidimensional event (Leenaars, 2004). Within the larger ecological frame, at the individual level, suicide is a state of existence, a human malaise, or condition, or pain. The suicide of our soldier/veteran has minimally the following intrapsychic (within the mind or psyche) characteristics: unbearable psychological pain, mental constriction (or distorted thinking), indirect expressions (such as dissembling), psychopathology (or inability to adjust), and a deep vulnerability (ego). He/she has at least the following interpersonal characteristics: traumatic problems in a relationship(s) (or towards an ideal, e.g., freedom, health, being a soldier), loss/rejection-aggression, and a need to escape (identification-egression). Beyond the psychological elements, and especially in a collective military culture, suicide has strong community and societal aspects. We should keep this system theory or conceptualization in mind as we improve care for our soldiers and veterans.

Suicide notes of soldiers

The best looking glass into the mind of the suicidal warrior is the suicide note.

A 21-year-old male soldier had traveled to Detroit to bury his mother, who died by overdose of pills. He wrote:

Mary
I'm sorry I had to do this, but I had no choice. After Mom died, I no longer had any reason to go on. I've just realized it.
I have no future and life is entirely pointless. I've been deceiving myself all along and its time it stopped.
On the train on the way back from Detroit to Fort Bragg, I thought of this. Returning to the stinking Army made me realize all I was doing was wasting another 3 years. And then what was I going to do? Well, there isn't any positive answer.
I love you all very much and was glad you and Sharon and Mike and the kids and I got together.
Love,
Bill

A 20-year-old male soldier, who had a physical disability resulting from an automobile accident, was distraught over the recent death of a close friend and said to his girlfriend that he was going to kill himself. Shortly thereafter, she broke up with him. He shot himself in the head with a .38 revolver. He wrote:

I loved her so much. I'm so sorry but this is how its gotta be. I hate life. Life's done me wrong. Please God forgive me but I'm weak. My lifes finished.

Keeping secrets

One final deadly point on suicide: Two or more out of ten suicidal people give no warning (Shneidman, 1985). The number is much higher in the armed forces. On secrecy, Captain Edwin Shneidman (1994) (he served as Captain in WWII, and worked for years at the VA) stated, "We suicidologists who deal with potentially suicidal people must....understand that in the ambivalent flow and flux of life, some desperately suicidal people....can dissemble and hide their true lethal feelings from the world" (p. 395).

Of course, people keep secrets. There are several types of secrets: supportive, protective, manipulative, and avoidant. The manipulative and avoidant secrets are a major cause of anxiety, PTSD, depression, and suicide risk. They are deadly, especially in the military. Soldiers and veterans often dissemble with fellow soldiers, parents, spouses, therapists, even sergeants.

Suicide among the U.S. Armed Forces

Durkheim (1897/1951) provided the earliest figures available on military suicide in the US; he reported a rate of 68 per 100,000 for the U.S. Army after the Civil War. This, to date, was a matchless epidemic of suicide among the U.S. forces. A high-risk group for suicide was the commanders; some of the greatest Civil War heroes and leaders, such as General Emory Upton, died by suicide. What are the wages of war? We know that throughout the 20th century, suicides as a cause of death within the U.S. military were second only to accidents. Even so, the suicide data has always been unreliable.

Surveillance is everything in public (system) health. Shneidman (1980) published a paper on the poor surveillance in the U.S. military decades ago; there was up to a 60% error in the count. A 2004 study found at least a 21% miscount. Therefore, we can conclude that suicides were and are underreported in the U.S. military.

What are the reported recent rates of U.S. military suicide? Opinion has become divided about whether U.S. military soldiers and veterans are at increased risk. In the early years of the Iraq and Afghanistan Wars, official confirmed U.S. soldier suicides were few. However, the rates in 2003 and 2005 were 18.8 and 19.9 per 100,000, respectively. This compares to around 11.6 suicides per 100,000 in the general population. Simply being in harm's way is risk; there is a cost of service. Military service has, in fact, now been accepted as a risk factor for suicide and suicidal behavior. There is a recent rise in the rate of suicide among active-duty military service personnel; according to Thompson (2012), one soldier dies by suicide per day.

What about veterans? Early, the official reports suggested low rates. However, the data were distorted. Kaplan, Huguet, McFarland, and Newson (2007) have, in fact, shown that U.S. military veterans are twice as likely to die by suicide as civilians. A major problem with earlier studies has been the reliance on the data from Department of Veterans Affairs (VA) system. Kaplan et al. note that:

> The reliance on VA clinical samples is particularly limiting from a population-based perspective because three-quarters of veterans do not receive healthcare through VA facilities. Consequently, little is known about the risk factors for suicide among veterans in the general U.S. population... In light of the high incidence of physical and mental disabilities among veterans of the conflicts in Iraq and Afghanistan ... it is important to examine the risk of suicide among veterans in the general population. (p. 619)

Kaplan and his team, in fact, examined the risk factors for suicide among veterans in the general population. The main outcome variable was death by suicide. Suicide cases were identified using The International Classification of Diseases, ninth revision, clinical modification (ICD-9 E950-3959). One key predictive variable was veteran status. Kaplan and his group's results were striking:

> Veterans represented 15.7% of the NHIS sample but accounted for 31.1% of the suicide decedents. Over time veterans were twice as likely (adjusted HR 2.13, 95% CI 1.14 to 3.99) to die of suicide compared with male non-veterans in the general population. Conversely, the risk of death from natural (diseases) and the risk of death from external (accidents and homicides) causes did not differ between the veterans and the non-veterans after we adjusted for confounding factors. (p. 620)

What were the predictors of suicide risk among veterans? "The results indicate that whites, those with > 12 years of education and those with activity limitations (after adjusting for medical and psychiatric morbidity) were at a greater risk for suicide completion" (p. 620). Kaplan et al. further state: "Veterans were at greater risk of dying from suicide compared with a non-veteran cohort. The results of this study are particularly noteworthy because they are derived from a sample representative of all veterans in the US general population, whether or not they sought care in the VA system" (p. 620).

They also noted a critical factor related to physical injuries. Many of these soldiers are limited in daily functioning, social skills, intellectual/memory functioning, or the ability to adjust. What else do we know? Almost always firearms were used. A common military belief is: "All soldiers die with their gun in hand." Soldiers and veterans are familiar with and know how to use a gun effectively. They have been trained to be deadly in the kill.

Posttraumatic Stress Disorder and suicide in the military

How does a soldier experience war-related events? Here is one soldier's story:

> Boom!...silence. Thank God we all survived, but my battle is not over. Since that battle I suffer from nightmares: I see the blood, I hear the screams. I am frustrated, I feel like a failure; nothing seems to interest me any longer. I have lost my ability to be happy. (Koren, Hilel, Idar, Hemel, and Klein, 2007, p. 119)

It has previously been argued that the aftermath of suicide and other trauma for survivors is best viewed from a posttraumatic stress framework (Leenaars and Wenckstern, 1991). Adjustment to trauma is complex. Janoff-Bulman (1992) noted that much of the psychological trauma produced by victimizing events derives from the shattering of very basic assumptions (or beliefs) that victims held about the operation of the world. Wilson, Smith, and Johnson (1985) highlighted that the victims of a traumatic event, such as war-related trauma or a suicide, may be stuck in a no-win cycle of events:

> To talk about the powerful and overwhelming trauma means risking further stigmatization; the failure to discuss the traumatic episode increases the need for defensive avoidance and thus

increases the probability of depression alternating with cycles of intensive imagery and other symptoms of PTSD. (p. 169)

War violates many core beliefs. Regrettably, after traumatic experiences, a common response in the military is, "Snap out of it," or "Just go on with your duty". However, avoidance only exacerbates the problem. It has been concluded from previous research on PTSD (Figley, 1985) that the type of response provided largely affects an individual's adjustment to a trauma, whether it is war-related or suicide.

Reports related to military personnel returning from Vietnam, and now Afghanistan and Iraq, suggest that there are significant rates of psychological problems among these veterans. There is a higher risk for suicide (Farberow, Kang, and Bullman, 1990). Traumatic Brain Injury (TBI) is especially noted as a huge risk factor, but also other physical injuries. Many of those wounded in Afghanistan and Iraq are surviving injuries that would have previously proven fatal. This is a perfect storm for PTSD. Any normal person would experience fear, horror, and helplessness.

Koren, Hilel, Idar, Hemel, and Klein (2007) studied the interplay between combat, physical injury, and psychological trauma. They found:

> First, the prevalence of PTSD among the injured group (16.7%) was approximately 7 times higher (!) than the prevalence of PTSD among the noninjured group (2.5%)....Similarly, although somewhat less dramatically, the prevalence of other psychiatric disorders (such as depression, drug abuse, and adjustment disorder) that developed after the traumatic event was 2 times higher among the injured participants (10%) than the noninjured ones (5%). (p. 126)

Obviously, the relation between the severity of the injury and the severity of the posttraumatic reaction is not a linear one. Koren et al. (2007) concluded that "the growing mass of research in the field of physical injury and posttraumatic reactions indicates that physical injury during a traumatic event is probably a risk factor, rather than a protective factor, in the development of PTSD" (p. 124). Thus, not only mental pain, but also physical injury, is a risk factor for the development of PTSD and suicide risk.

Sadly, we also know that returning veterans may not be availing themselves of mental health treatment. In a military culture, a warrior does not get help. However, there are also many veterans, living with mental or physical unbearable pain, and a sense of hopelessness-helplessness, who continue to call for more acceptance, help, psychotherapy, financial stability, and honor. Too little is done, they state. Maybe, it is not only about soldiers and veterans availing themselves of help, but also availability of service. This is especially so for veterans with mental illness; veterans are quoted as stating that "the criteria are arbitrary, the funds insufficient" for help. Too many soldiers and veterans are left on the mental battlefield; the everlasting howling of the bombs and the deadly screams from seriously injured and dying never go away. Ask any veteran: there is understandable shell shock.

Secondary traumatization: Families, spouses, and children

The families of traumatized soldiers and veterans are indirect victims of their traumatic experience. This is called secondary traumatization (Dekel and Solomon, 2007). Combat stress injury has many victims and there are many faces of the aftershocks; PTSD spreads. Wives, children, parents, and even friends can become victims and casualties. Wives of veterans have described PTSD symptoms, including dreams of the war and panic attacks triggered by the same triggers as their husband's, such as the buzz of helicopters, sudden noises, and gunfire (Dekel and Solomon, 2007). One wife has described surviving her husband's war stress as "walking on eggshells."

There is, of course, considerable variance in the adjustment of spouses of veterans. PTSD severity is associated with multiple factors; many echo the ones that place soldiers at risk. Indeed, the soldier's PTSD predicts the secondary traumatization. Avoidance symptoms especially affect the quality of the marital relationship. Consistent with domestic violence literature, the more frequent the violence of a military husband suffering from PTSD toward his wife, the higher the wife's distress. These observations seem obvious, and there have been some theoretical explanations; the one most consistent with the evidence is identification and empathy. As with PTSD in soldiers and veterans, Janoff-Bulman (1992) suggests that the spouses' and families' world assumptions or beliefs are blown apart.

> This is that just as the basic world assumptions of direct victims of trauma are often upset (Janoff-Bulman, 1992), so too are the assumptions of indirect victims. The partner of a traumatized man

> learns, just as he had, that the world is unsafe and chaotic and that
> being a good person does not protect one from harm. Her basic
> assumptions about the relationship are also upset. (Dekel and
> Solomon, 2007, p. 149)

It is, of course, not only the spouse, but also the children who suffer from the combat friction. Sometimes, these children become orphans of the war, so the friction has secondary traumatization. The sudden death of a military parent is tragic, but it is not the only trauma. Children of military parents, of course, encounter potential traumatic experiences as any child (e.g., fires, car accidents). Yet, certain unique, traumatic events can pose risks to military children, such as a combat or non-combat (i.e., accidental) death. Suicide, of course, given the high rate, is one more increased probable traumatization.

Whether suicide or otherwise, the deaths are very real for children of military personnel; they are understandably traumatized. Friction continues, especially given a sudden and horrific death such as by improvised explosive device (IED) or accident. This is even more so if a death is by suicide. Like their military parent(s), the children feel shame and disgrace. These children are stressed and overwhelmed by emotions and reactions. Yet, we must not forget: Soldiers, veterans, and their military families, including the children, are typically resilient, as are most people. Despite the unbearable pain, grievers can count on their strengths, but outside support is critical.

Surviving suicide in the Armed Forces

> A person's death is not only an ending; it is also a beginning – for
> the survivors. Indeed, in the case of suicide, the largest public
> health problem is neither the prevention of suicide… nor the
> management of attempts… but the alleviation of the effects of
> stress in the survivor-victims of suicidal deaths, whose lives are
> forever changed….(Shneidman, 1973, p. 33)

How do survivors adjust to one of the worst possible traumas that occurs in a war, a suicide? One fact is absolute: The pain of the suicide becomes the pain of the survivor. Anguish, guilt, anger, sadness, shame, dishonor, and anxiety are a sample of the pains. They have a haunting existence. Arnold Toynbee (1968) makes the point that death is a two-party event. He writes:

The two-sidedness of death is a fundamental feature of death—not only of the premature death of the spirit, but also of death at any age and in any form. There are always two parties to a death; the person who dies and the survivors who are bereaved...

The sting of death is less sharp for the person who dies than it is for the bereaved survivor.

This, as I see it, is the capital fact about the relation between living and dying. There are two parties to the suffering that death inflicts; and in the apportionment of this suffering, the survivor takes the brunt. (pp. 327-332)

Toynbee here resonates to Saint Paul's question, "O death, where is thy sting?" The brunt is even more for the survivors of suicide in the military. This suffering is even greater than expected of war, the inflicting more intentional. There is frequently a belief that the sting was malicious. Survivors of a soldier's or veteran's suicide may ask, "Did he (or she) want me to hurt so?" There can be complicated grief.

Suicide is a dyadic event. It is a relationship, and especially in a collective culture, also a deep community and societal event. Shneidman (1972) noted:

I believe that the person who commits suicide puts his psychological skeletons in the survivor's emotional closet – he sentences the survivor – to deal with many negative feelings and, more, to become obsessed with thoughts regarding his own actual or possible role in having precipitated the suicidal act or having failed to abort it. It can be a heavy load. (p. 10)

It is significant that the "extent of the problem" of suicide survivorship in the general population has only been recognized in the last 15 to 20 years. There has been a rapidly growing effort by many professionals, psychologists, social workers, psychiatrists, nurses, and the lay public to understand the "skeletons." Yet, there are still taboos and walls, and these have been shown to be even more so in the military (Leenaars, 2013).

PRINCIPLES OF POSTVENTION

How will the soldier's or veteran's suicide affect the lives of family, friends, fellow soldiers, health providers, and the public? Prevention, intervention, and postvention in the armed forces are imperative in addressing the public health crisis of suicide among soldiers and veterans. Prevention is, in fact, a mandatory response of a caring, humanistic institution. *Postvention*, a term introduced by Shneidman (1973, 1975), refers to those things done after the event has occurred. Postvention deals with the traumatic aftereffects in the survivors of a person who died by suicide (or in those close to someone who has attempted suicide). Postvention in suicide involves offering mental health and public health services to the bereaved survivors. Family, friends, fellow soldiers, local service providers, and so on, may need help in the loss and grief. Postvention includes improving care with all survivors who are in need.

Shneidman (1975) had provided us with some principles of postvention, which are common, in responding to the postsuicide event. They are largely based on his extensive work with survivors in a psychotherapeutic context. The following principles of postvention are derived from Shneidman but have been liberally modified for application to any trauma within the military or other system (e.g., a school setting) (Leenaars and Wenckstern, 1998)·

1. In working with survivor victims of suicide, it is best to begin as soon as possible after the tragedy, within the first 24 hours if that can be managed.
2. Resistance may be met from the survivors; some, but not all, may be willing to have the opportunity to talk to professionally oriented persons.
3. Negative emotions about the decedent (the deceased person) or about any trauma—irritation, anger, fear, shame, guilt, and so on—need to be explored, but not at the very beginning. Timing is so important.
4. The postventionist should play the important role of reality tester. He/she is not so much the echo of conscience as the quiet voice of reason.
5. One should be constantly alert for possible decline in health and in overall mental well-being, especially suicide risk.
6. Needless to say, overt optimism or banal platitudes should be avoided.
7. Trauma work is multifaceted and takes a while—from several months to the end of life, but certainly more than 90 minutes.
8. A comprehensive program of healthcare on the part of a benign and enlightened community should include prevention, intervention, and postvention.

Policies and procedures from the military

One of the best documents focusing on recommendations for postvention is from the Department of the Army (2009), *Suicide postvention. Health promotion, risk reduction, and suicide prevention.*

Postvention
4–1. General

Postvention consists of a sequence of planned support and interventions carried out with survivors in the aftermath of a completed suicide or suicide attempt. Postvention is prevention for survivors. The goal of suicide postvention is to support those affected by a suicide or attempt, promote healthy recovery, reduce the possibility of suicide contagion, strengthen unit cohesion, and promote continued mission readiness.

a. When implementing a Postvention program, commanders will do the following:

(1) Provide long term support to Families, unit members, and co-workers who experience loss due to suicide. Care can be provided via external services and outreach programs including civilian services for grief and recovery (that is, Department of Veterans Affairs Bereavement Counseling, Tragedy Assistance Program for Survivors (TAPS), Survivor Outreach Services [SOS])...

(2) Postvention activities include unit-level interventions following an attempted or completed suicidal in order to minimize psychological reactions to the event, prevent or minimize the potential for copy cat suicides, strengthen unit cohesion, and promote continued mission readiness...

(3) Provide care to the friends of someone who has attempted or completed suicide. The command must proactively address the situation and provide an outlet for those affected to express and process their emotions...

4–2. Army suicide behavior surveillance

Army suicide behavior surveillance is a critical postvention activity, which includes the collection of informational data about suicide behavior by all components...

b. Psychological autopsies may be requested by the Armed Forces Medical Examiner (AFME) and/or the Criminal Investigation Command (CID) on Active Duty deaths under special circumstances, in accordance with AR 600–63, paragraph 4–4. Additionally, the senior commander may request a psychological autopsy through CID. The psychological autopsy is a forensic investigative tool that is used to confirm or refute the death of an individual by suicide. It is not to be confused with gathering of information for suicide event surveillance for epidemiological purposes. Specifically, psychological autopsies assist in ascertaining the manner of death; and will primarily be used to resolve cases where there is an equivocal cause of death; that is, death cannot be readily established as natural, accidental, a suicide, or a homicide. (p. 16-17)

Some thoughts on counseling military survivors

On the surface, common sense says that doing intensive postvention work with a survivor whose spouse, parent, or buddy died by suicide is different from working therapeutically with any other kind of person. In addition, if the person was a soldier or veteran, there are even more distinct factors. In grieving, the essential focus is not the death, but the survivor's emotional state of mind; the reality that one's loved one killed him or herself. Understandably, there are enormous feelings, thoughts, and consequences in that enduring situation. Psychologically, it is a deep "sting," deeper than the mind was aware of. Any sane person would respond with fear, horror, and helplessness.

There is an important difference that needs to be identified and addressed when working with a survivor, beyond the ordinary use of psychotherapy or counseling. The exchange between two people is a unique existential event. The very nature is a human exchange, one of whom (the survivor) is struggling with the suicide and the other (counselor), who is not surviving such a death (at least not proximally); but both are going to share the common factors of adjusting to the skeletons. That fact itself sets working with a survivor apart from usual psychotherapy or counseling.

Second, I believe it is anodynic, if the survivor develops a rather strong positive alliance toward the clinician who is seeking to help with the traumatic experience. The death may result in abundant (historical and current) reactions, distorted beliefs, and painful feelings. Negative reactions, such as feelings of anger, shame, or hopelessness, may arise. Of course, there is also the probability that countertransferences, the counselor's own reactions, thoughts and feelings, may come up. The importance is not what occurred, but how it is handled. There are many grief counselors working with military survivors who suffer secondary traumatization; a few, we know, have killed themselves too in this war.

A counselor must believe that the suicidal soldier, who served in harm's way, was not weak, limited, immature, or premorbidly aggressive. He or she was a "good soldier," but one who avoided seeking help in stressful situations. The veterans do not differ; few go to the VA, for example. Psychotherapy or counseling is rarely sought. This is equally true of the survivors from a military system. If a therapist does not hold to this core belief, it would be best that he/she does not treat suicidal soldiers or veterans or survivors of military suicide.

A final point: Despite one military personnel dying from suicide every day, military suicide is still a rare event statistically. The embedded fact is that the majority of soldiers and veterans are resilient. Meichenbaum (2012) reported that about 30% are too traumatized to be so. Seventy percent of the military personnel are resilient; but the other 30% simply need support. And suicide is only one example of the specter of war-related deaths that occur. Therefore, there is a host of survivors of different military deaths that a clinician will meet.

Most important in all of these situations is the therapeutic relationship. Grief counseling is concerned with what type of person the survivor is. Our grief counseling should address the person's story, his/her narrative, not the demographic, nosological category of this or that finding. Of course, the practical disadvantage of this approach is that it requires more than 90 minutes. Debriefing has, in fact, been debunked; it actually causes harm. Suicide postvention is not an efficiency operation. It is a human exchange.

Suicide postvention is based on a humanitarian approach to life. The psychotherapy or counseling that works best with survivors of suicide is a person-centered therapy, or a survivor-centered therapy, not mental disorder-centered therapy. The relationship should be what Martin Buber called an "I-Thou," not an "I-it." The relationship, attachment, or bond that the therapist develops is central in effective psychotherapy with survivors. Research shows that what works with survivors is, in fact, clearly associated to the helping relationship itself. What we have known for a long time is that survivors who persevere and benefit from psychotherapy are the ones that have developed a good working relationship or alliance. Empathy is imperative when counseling a survivor. Without empathy, one cannot, in fact, really work with another person.

Finally, what is the best person-centered counseling for survivors? Like me, reviewers in the field argue that there is no satisfactory objective data which allow us to state the "best." Indeed, many therapies can be helpful and sting-removing: Cognitive Behavioral Therapy, Anodyne Therapy, Psychodynamic, Dialectical-Behavioral Therapy, Person-Centered Therapy, Solution-Focused, among others.

It is also true that at times the postvention for an individual has to be multi-component and multi-disciplinary. It has, in fact, been concluded that multi-component interventions in military personnel probably reduce the risk of suicide best. To present the knowledge is beyond the scope of this paper (Leenaars, 2004). I will, however, note some challenges to implement a strategy for postvention with an armed forces population. We may need to look at medication, hospitalization (which may be rarely necessary, and should always be implemented with caution), and environmental control (gun control is always a must). However, I am inclined to believe that psychotherapy or counseling with survivors is most helpful. Fortunately, we have abundant healers beyond Shneidman (1972, 1973, 1975) who can guide us. The American Association of Suicidology (www.suicidology.org), founded by Shneidman in 1968, is an excellent resource for finding trained professionals and support materials.

The goals in grief counseling are typically limited; full psychological health is not the objective. The goal is to make the dire situation go as well as possible; to accept the unacceptable; and to go on living with the death. The counselor needs to trust the survivor's military courage. Courage is the ability to change what one can. The anodynic experience, to somewhat quote Aldous Huxley, is not what happened to the survivor, it is what he or she does with what happened. The survivor needs to trust her or his hardiness. Despite all that has happened to him/her, the military, the war, the suicide, beyond what was imagined by the soldier (since the first day he or she went to boot camp) and the survivor, the survivor can adjust. The major reframing in counseling: You can survive the unbearable pain.

Suicide is seldom a uni-person event. There is a community at risk; this is especially so in the military's collective society. It follows that postvention with a survivor ought almost always include more than one person. No postvention with military survivors can be isolated; postvention may include the commander, family members, fellow veterans or soldiers, friends, or minister. It takes the military community to survive all war-related deaths. This is consistent with the WHO's (2002) ecological model for treatment.

Typically, grief counseling is enough, although not always. The grief counselor needs always to be aware of the aftershocks. Some, not all, may need to be in more traditional therapy.

Some very distinct military factors

The main obstacle to help-seeking in the military is the negative attitude towards doing so. There are enormous unique barriers to getting help. The military's own researchers (Ritchie, Keppler, and Rothberg, 2003) stated that this is because in the past, people in the armed forces were not talking about what was happening. There were suicides; however, the deaths were kept secret. The main reason, the military professionals stated, was stigma. It was not acceptable to be suicidal, or to get help; somehow it was more acceptable to lie in a coffin. The U.S. military is now intent on changing this iatrogenic attitude.

The first big step is accepting the problem. Institutions and individuals must be organized strategically for suicide prevention, and leaders must be supportive at every level. The U.S. military is beginning to recognize the many faces of traumatization of war; PTSD and suicide risk are just two possible aftershocks. The U.S. military must accept the secondary traumatization of the family; everyone can feel the friction.

There are further barriers; one factor is limited access to mental health services. Most survivors call for more help; however, in the military's collective society, survivors may feel estranged and disenfranchised. As in the greater society, there is a prejudicial view, if you die by suicide, you are not a hero. There has been such shame and disgrace about mental health and suicide risk in the military. To treat survivors, and for that matter, soldiers and veterans, effectively, this wall has to come down.

Treatment of suicide survivors among the armed forces cannot work without an atmosphere of trust. However, many military families are reluctant to get help; many fear what they say in counseling at the VA, for example, will not be private. Survivors believe that they cannot be honest. This has to change if we are even able to counsel military survivors.

To date, there exists no significant body of literature identifying specific concerns and areas of the unique challenges for helping survivors in the military. Therefore, more research and information on military postvention is needed.

A CALL TO DUTY

The military needs to ask some tough questions: Who are war-related deaths? What are the painful short and long-term consequences of war trauma for the armed services members and veterans? Why does suicide occur epidemically? What are life-saving military factors? What are the barriers to wellness in the military? What can be done to more effectively care for our at-risk-for-suicide warriors and veterans? What can we do for survivors if suicide occurs? How can we improve care? What can we do to improve postvention? Furthermore, of course, in light of current high rates of military suicide in America, there is the dire question: Will we continue to allow our soldiers and veterans to suffer the unbearable friction and die by their own hands?

Antoon A. Leenaars, Ph.D., C.Psych., CPQ, is a psychologist in private practice in mental health and public health in Windsor, Canada, and is senior advisor at The Norwegian Institute of Public Health, Oslo, Norway. He was the first past president of the Canadian Association for Suicide Prevention (CASP) and a past president of the American Association of Suicidology (AAS), the only non-American. He is author/editor of Psychotherapy with Suicidal People, Suicide among the Armed Forces, *and 11 additional books, as well as over 230 articles and chapters. He was the founding Editor-in-Chief of the journal* Archives of Suicide Research. *Dr. Leenaars is a recipient of the International Association for Suicide Prevention's Erwin Stengel Award, CASP's Research Award, and AAS's Edwin Shneidman Award. He has consulted to the WHO, institutions and governments around the world and has provided forensic services in cases of wrongful death, suicide, homicide-suicide, and homicide for police services, and legal institutions.*

References

Christian, J., Stivers, J., & Sammons, M. (2009). Training to the warrior ethos: Implications for clinicians treating military members and their families. In S. Freeman, B. Moore, & A. Freeman (Eds.), *Living and surviving in harm's way* (pp. 27-49). New York, NY: Routledge.

Dekel, R., & Solomon, Z. (2007). Secondary traumatization among wives of war veterans with PTSD. In C. Figley & W. Nash (Eds.), *Combat stress injury* (pp. 137-157). New York, NY: Routledge.

Department of the Army. (2009). *Health promotion, risk reduction, and suicide prevention.* Washington, DC: Author.

Durkheim, E. (1951). *Suicide.* (Translated by J. Spaulding & G. Simpson). London, England: Routledge & Kegan Paul. (Original published in 1897).

Farberow, N., Kang, H., & Bullman, T. (1990). Combat experience and postservice psychosocial status as predictors of suicide in Vietnam Veterans. *The Journal of Nervous and Mental Disease, 178,* 32-37.

Figley, C. (Ed.) (1985). *Trauma and its wake.* New York, NY: Brunner/Mazel.

Hall, L. (2011). The military culture, language, and lifestyle. In R. Everson & C. Figley (Eds.), *Families under fire* (pp. 31-52). New York, NY: Routledge.

Janoff-Bulman, R. (1992). *Shattered assumptions: Towards a new psychology of trauma.* New York, NY: The Free Press.

Kaplan, M., Huguet, N., McFarland, B., & Newsom, J. (2007) Suicide among male veterans: a prospective population-based study. *Journal of Epidemiology and Community Health, 61,* 619-624.

Koren, D., Hilel, Y., Idar, N., Hemel, E., & Klein, E. (2007). Combat stress management: The interplay between combat, physical injury, and psychological trauma. In C. Figley & W. Nash (Eds.), *Combat stress injury* (pp. 119-135). New York, NY: Routledge.

Leenaars, A. (2004). *Psychotherapy with suicidal people: A person-centered approach.* Chichester, England: John Wiley & Sons.

Leenaars, A. (2007). Suicide: A cross-cultural theory. In F. Leong & M. Leach (Eds.), *Suicide among racial and ethnic minority groups* (pp. 13-37). New York, NY: Routledge.

Leenaars, A. (2013). *Suicide among the Armed Forces: Understanding the cost of service.* Amityville, NY: Baywood.

Leenaars, A., & Wenckstern, S. (1991). Posttraumatic stress disorder: A conceptual model for postvention. In A. Leenaars & S. Wenckstern (Eds.), *Suicide prevention in schools* (pp. 173-195). Washington, DC: Hemisphere Publishing Corporation.

Leenaars, A., & Wenckstern, S. (1998). Principles of postvention. *Death Studies, 22,* 357-391.

Meichenbaum, D. (2012). *Road map to resilience: A guide for military, trauma victims, and their families.* Clearwater, FL: Institute Press.

Ritchie, E., Keppler, W., & Rothberg, J. (2003). Suicidal admissions in the United States military. *Military Medicine, 168,* 177-181.

Shneidman, E. (1972). Foreword. In A. Cain (Ed.), *Survivors of suicide* (pp. ix-xi). Springfield, IL: Charles C. Thomas.

Shneidman, E. (1973). *Deaths of man.* New York, NY: Quadrangle.

Shneidman, E. (1975). Postvention: Care of the bereaved. In R. Pasnau (Ed.), *Consultation-liaison psychiatry* (pp. 245-256). New York, NY: Grune & Stratton.

Shneidman, E. (1980). The reliability of suicide statistics: A bomb-burst. *Suicide & Life-Threatening Behavior, 10,* 67-69.

Shneidman, E. (1985). *Definition of suicide.* New York, NY: John Wiley & Sons.

Shneidman, E. (1994). Clues to suicide reconsidered. *Suicide & Life-Threatening Behavior, 24,* 395-397.

Thompson, M. (2012, June). U.S. Military suicides in 2012:155 days, 154 dead. *Time.* Retrieved October 2012 from http://nation.time.com/2012/06/08/lagging-indicator/

Toynbee, A. (1968). Man's concern with death. New York, NY: McGraw-Hill. Quoted in E. Shneidman (Ed.). (1973). *Death: Current perspectives*. Palo Alto, CA: Mayfield Publishing Co.

Wilson, J., Smith, W., & Johnson, S. (1985). A comparative analysis of PTSD among various survivor groups. In C. Figley (Ed.), *Trauma and its wake* (pp. 142-172). New York, NY: Brunner/Mazel.

World Health Organization (WHO) (2002). *World report on violence and health*. Geneva: Author.

Concluding Comments

Kenneth J. Doka

The American Soldier Study (Stouffer et al., 1949) began as a study of how to best recruit, train, motivate, and reintegrate soldiers in World War II. It had import far beyond those initial goals. Concepts that derived from the study such as relative deprivation and anticipatory socialization, as well as methodological techniques developed for the study, enriched the fields of sociology and social psychology immeasurably.

In a similar vein, as we assist veterans in facing illness and death, the lessons learned may have import far beyond veterans. For example, the culture of stoicism, while amplified in the military, is widely shared among many segments of American society. One of the major impediments to effective pain management is sometimes called the Dubose Syndrome, named after Mrs. Dubose, a character in the classic American novel *To Kill a Mockingbird* by Harper Lee. After having been a morphine addict for years, Mrs. Dubose chooses to die without the use of opioids (Doka, 2006). For many individuals the ability to withstand pain is a mark of courage and character.

This model of extrapolating medical knowledge from veterans' experiences can be seen in current situations with veterans from more recent wars. Many Vietnam veterans were exposed to Agent Orange, and managing the symptoms and illnesses related to this has raised awareness of the diseases associated with chemical exposure. Treatment of the injuries sustained by many veterans from the wars in Iraq and Afghanistan, such as traumatic brain injuries and amputations, has impacted treatment for non-veterans dealing with these same issues.

The use of marijuana and other substances including prescription medication was not just an aspect of military culture but generally shared through the Baby Boomer Generation. Hence the lessons we learn about pain assessment and management will have wider value.

In addition veterans were not the only population that experienced traumatic events. Such experiences are shared by police, firefighters, other first responders, and individuals who experienced or witnessed traumatic events. The lessons learned about life review and Posttraumatic Stress Disorder once again will have more extensive import.

Though that is likely the case, we need to reaffirm that in the end it is a secondary benefit. Effective end-of-life care for veterans facing illness and death is a value in and of itself. It is not a gift but a right earned by service and sacrifice.

REFERENCES

Doka, K.J. (2006). Social, cultural, spiritual, and psychological barriers to pain management. In K. Doka (Ed.), *Pain management at the end-of-life: Bridging the gap between knowledge and practice.* (pp. 59-73). Washington, DC: The Hospice Foundation of America.

Stouffer, S., Lumsdaine, R., Harper, M., Smith, M., Janis, I., Star, S., and Cottrell, L. (1949). *The American soldier: Combat and its aftermath,* (V-4). Princeton, NJ: Princeton University Press.

Resources

Listed below are some helpful grief and veteran-related websites and organizations, many of which were referenced by the authors.

Grief Resources:
- American Widow Project, www.americanwidowproject.org
- Association for Death Education and Counseling (ADEC), www.adec.org
- The Compassionate Friends (TCF), www.compassionatefriends.org
- National Alliance for Grieving Children, www.childrengrieve.org
- National Widowers' Organization, www.nationalwidowers.org
- Young Widow, www.youngwidow.org

Veteran Resources:
- Department of Veterans Affairs, www.va.gov
  This website offers a wide range of information for veterans, including Veteran's Benefits Administration, CHAMPVA, data on veterans, and VHA Forms and Publications.
- Vet Centers, www.vetcenter.va.gov
- To obtain bereavement counseling, www.vetcenter.va.gov or call 202-461-6530
- The American Legion, www.legion.org
- Dignity Memorial, www.dignitymemorial.com
- Military OneSource, www.militaryonesource.com
- National Cemetery Administration, www.cem.va.gov
- National Center for PTSD, www.ptsd.va.gov
- Tragedy Assistance Program for Survivors (TAPS), www.taps.org
- TRICARE, www.tricare.mil
- USO, www.uso.org
- VA Caregiver Support, www.caregiver.va.gov
- Vietnam Veterans of America, www.vva.org

- Veterans Crisis Line, www.veteranscrisisline.net or 1-800-273-8255
- Veterans of Foreign Wars, www.vfw.org
- We Honor Veterans, www.wehonorveterans.org

Military Family Resources:
- American Gold Star Mothers, Inc., www.goldstarmoms.com
- Give-An-Hour, www.giveanhour.org
- Gold Star Wives of America, Inc., www.goldstarwives.org
- Got Your Back Network, www.gotyourbacknetwork.org
- Hope for the Warriors, www.hopeforthewarriors.org
- Military Families United, www.militaryfamiliesunited.org
- National Military Family Association, www.nmfa.org
- Snowball Express, www.snowballexpress.org
- Travis Manion Foundation, www.travismanion.org

Professional Resources:
- End-of-Life Nursing Education Consortium (ELNEC), part of the American Association of College of Nursing (AACN), www.aacn.nche.edu/elnec
- EPEC: Education in Palliative and End-of-Life Care, www.epec.net
- Hospice and Palliative Nurses Association (HPNA), www.hpna.org
- Military History Pocket Card for Clinicians, www.va.gov/oaa/pocketcard
- *Wounded Warriors: Their Last Battle*, Facilitator's Guide for Grief Work with Veterans' Families, www.wehonorveterans.org
- Language Translations for Wong Baker's Faces Pain Scale, http://www.wongbakerfaces.org/public_html/wp-content/uploads/2012/02/10Translations.pdf

Print Resources:
- *Peace at Last: Stories of Hope and Healing for Veterans and their Families* by Deborah Grassman
- *The Hero Within: Redeeming the Destiny We were Born to Fulfill* by Deborah Grassman

The Military History Checklist that follows was developed through a collaborative effort of the NHPCO Veterans Advisory Council and the VA Hospice and Palliative Care Program. The questions are based on the VA Office of Academic Affiliations' (OAA) Military Service History Pocket Card (www.va.gov/oaa).

MILITARY HISTORY CHECKLIST

PATIENT DATA	Completed By:	
Patient's Name:	Date:	
Address:	Hospice Medical Record #:	Last 4 SSN:

VETERAN STATUS INFORMATION

1. Did you (or your spouse or family member) serve in the military?

1a. Patient ☐Yes ☐No	Did you serve on active duty?	☐Yes ☐No
	Did your service include combat, dangerous or traumatic assignments?	☐Yes ☐No
	Do you have a copy of your DD214 discharge papers?	☐Yes ☐No

1b. Did your spouse serve on active duty? ☐Yes ☐No
Comments:

1c. Do you have any immediate family members that served or are serving in the military? ☐Yes ☐No
Comments:

MILITARY BACKGROUND

2. In which branch of the military did you serve?

☐Army	☐Marines	☐Merchant Marines during WWII
☐Navy	☐Coast Guard	☐Other _____
☐Air Force	☐Reservist or National Guard member	

3. In which war era or period of service did you serve?

☐WWI (4/6/17 to 11/11/18)	☐Vietnam (8/5/64 to 5/7/75 and 2/28/61 for Veterans who served "in country" (in Vietnam) before 8/5/64)	☐Peace Time
☐WWII (12/7/41 to 12/31/46)		☐Afghanistan/Iraq (OEF/OIF)
☐Korea (6/27/50 to 1/31/55)		☐Other
☐Cold War	☐Gulf War (8/2/90 through a date to be set by law or presidential proclamation)	Note: after 9/7/80, must have completed 24 months continuous active service, or the full period for which they were called or ordered to active duty.

4. Overall, how do you view your experience in the military?

5. If available would you like your hospice staff/volunteer to have military experience? ☐Yes ☐No

VA BENEFITS INFORMATION

6. Are you enrolled in VA? ☐Yes ☐No

6a. Do you receive any VA benefits? ☐Yes ☐No

6b. Do you have a service-connected condition? ☐Yes ☐No

6c. Do you get your medications from VA? ☐Yes ☐No

6d. What is the name of your VA hospital or clinic?

6e. What is the name and contact information of your VA physician or Primary Care Provider?

6f. Would you like to talk with someone about benefits you or your family might be eligible to receive? ☐Yes ☐No

Index

A

Acetaminophen, 118

Active-duty deaths, 185, 213–217. *See also* Combat deaths

Affirmation rituals, 167

Afghanistan War
    culture of combat, 28–29
    demographics of surviving families, 191–192
    demographics of the deceased, 190–191
    statistics from, 27

AFME. *See* Armed Forces Medical Examiner

African Americans
    Traditionalists, 49

Age cohorts, 47–52

Agent Orange
    diagnosing medical conditions, 40–43

Alcoholics Anonymous, 117

ALS. *See* Amyotrophic lateral sclerosis

American Association of Suicidology, 233

American Gold Star Mothers, Inc., 207

American Legion, 10, 90, 142–143

American Sociological Association, 47

American Soldier Study, 241

American Widow Project, 207

Amyotrophic lateral sclerosis, 52

Anger, 105–107

Anodyne therapy, 232

Antidepressants, 119–120

Armed Forces Medical Examiner, 231

Army Survivor Outreach Services Program, 200, 207

Association for Death Education and Counseling, 205

B

Baby Boomer Generation, 49, 50–52

Bad-conduct discharges, 144

"Battle fatigue," 72

Bereaved Family Survey, 145–146

Bereavement counseling, 90–91. *See also* Grief

BFS. *See* Bereaved Family Survey

Breakthrough pain, 119

Burials
    burial benefits, 34
    combat deaths and, 200–201

Bush, George W., 171

Byock, Ira, 184

C

CACO. *See* Casualty Assistance Call Officers

CAICC. *See* Center for Advanced Illness Coordinated Care

CAO. *See* Casualty Assistance Officers

Capsaicin, 118

Caregiver services, 179–180

Caregiver Support Coordinators, 180

Casualty Assistance Call Officers, 199–200

Casualty Assistance Officers, 199–200

Catastrophic Coverage directive, 139

CBOCs. *See* Community Based Outpatient Clinics

CBT. *See* Cognitive-behavioral therapy

CELC. *See* Comprehensive End-of-Life Care

Cemeteries
    National Cemetery Administration, 136
    role in grief and loss, 161

Center for Advanced Illness Coordinated Care, 66

Central Office, Department of Veterans Affairs, 59–60

Central pain, 111

CHAMPVA, 180

Checklist, Military History, 52, 144, 245

Children. *See also* Families
    effects of military service, 5–6
    secondary traumatization, 226–227

Chronic Sorrow: A Living Loss, 179

CID. *See* Criminal Investigation Command

CLCs. *See* Community Living Centers

Cognitive-behavioral therapy, 117

247

Combat deaths. *See also* Active-duty deaths
  Casualty Officers, 199–200
  circumstances of death, 197–198
  death during deployment, 196–197
  death notification, 198–199
  demographics of surviving families, 191–192
  demographics of the deceased, 190–191
  funerals, memorials, and burials, 200–201
  grief process, 192–195
  immediate impact to survivors, 201
  impact on families, 189–190, 192–207
  media attention, 202
  political protestors, 202

Community Based Outpatient Clinics, 34, 90, 138

Community hospice agencies
  collaboration among, 139–143
  communication among, 136–139
  coordination among, 143–146
  creating a veteran-centric culture, 134–136
  Hospice-Veteran Partnerships, 133–147
  quality improvement, 145–146
  veteran-specific education curricula, 145

Community Living Centers, 62

Comprehensive End-of-Life Care, 68

Continuity rituals, 166

Control
  stoicism and, 12–13

Corticosteroid injections, 118

Counseling services, 79–80, 90–91

County Veteran Service Officers, 142–143

Courage
  confusion with stoicism, 12

Covenant Hospice, 152–153

Criminal Investigation Command, 231

Cultural issues. *See* Military culture

D

DAV. *See* Disabled American Veterans

Death. *See* Active-duty deaths; Combat deaths

Death notification, 198–199

Decedent Affairs Clerk, 178

Deployment-delayed grief, 197

Depression. *See also* Posttraumatic Stress Disorder; Suicide
  chronic pain and, 119–120
  refusal of treatment, 12

Details Clerk, 178

Diclofenac gel, 118

Disabled American Veterans, 10, 90

Dishonorable discharges, 144

Dissembling, 220

Dissociation, 120

The Dougy Center, 201

Drug abuse
  Posttraumatic Stress Disorder and, 116

Dubose Syndrome, 241

Duloxetine, 120

Dying Well, 184

E

Ecological fallacy, 47

Ecological model, 220

Education, veteran-specific, 145

Education in Palliative and End-of-Life Care, 145

ELNEC. *See* End-of-Life Nursing Education Consortium

ELNEC-for-Veterans, 145

EMDR. *See* Eye Movement Desensitization and Reprocessing

End-of-Life Nursing Education Consortium, 145

EPEC. *See* Education in Palliative and End-of-Life Care

EPEC for Veterans Project, 145

Ethos Consulting Group, 66

Exercise therapy, 117

Eye Movement Desensitization and Reprocessing, 206

F

Faces Pain Scale, 112

Faculty Leaders Project, 64

Families
  caregiver services, 179–180
  demographics of survivors, 191–192
  effects of military service, 5–6
  grief services for, 175–186
  impact of combat deaths, 189–190, 192–207
  impact of suicide, 226–227
  interventional strategies, 206–207
  military widows, 213–217
  resources, 243–244
  secondary traumatization, 226–227
  understanding veterans' inability to grieve, 180–181

Family Evaluation of Hospice Care-Veterans, 145–146

Family Program and Services, 207

Family Readiness Officers, 197

Federal Benefits for Veterans, Dependents and Survivors, 144

FEHC-V. *See* Family Evaluation of Hospice Care-Veterans

Fentanyl, 122

Financial issues, 179

Flag presentation, 178

Forgiveness, 95–101

The Forgotten War. *See* Korean War

"Friendly fire," 9, 96

FROs. See Family Readiness Officers

Funerals
    combat deaths and, 200–201
    disruption of, 171–172, 202
    enhancing the value of, 164–165
    therapeutic value of, 162–164

G

GEC. *See* Office of Geriatrics and Extended Care

Generational cohorts, 47–52

G.I. Bill. *See* Servicemen's Readjustment Act of 1944

GI Generation, 48–49

GI toxicity, 118–119

Gold Star Wives of America, Inc., 207

Graeber, Dr. Mark, 61

Grassman, Deborah, 105, 177, 181

Greater Los Angeles Health Care System, 61

The Greatest Generation. *See* World War II

Grief
    active-duty deaths and, 185
    bereavement counseling, 90–91
    combat deaths and, 192–207
    context of grieving prior to traumatic events, 86–89
    counseling services, 90–91
    counseling suicide survivors, 231–234
    disenfranchised grief, 205
    family services, 175–186
    interrelationship with trauma, 86–90
    loss and, 157–158
    military widows, 213–217
    Posttraumatic Stress Disorder and, 182–183
    resources, 243
    role of rituals and memorials, 161–168
    as the root of traumatic stress, 89–90
    stoicism and, 175, 181–182
    supporting veteran grief, 181–185
    veterans' inability to grieve, 180–181

Guilt, 95–98, 105–107

Gulf War
    noncombat military deaths, 11

H

Hand-heart connection, 100–101, 106–107

HBPC. *See* Home-Based Primary Care

HCFA. *See* Health Care Financing Administration

Health Care Financing Administration, 59

HEN. *See* Hospice Education Network

Home-Based Primary Care, 34, 138

Homeless veterans, 135

Honor Flight, 99

Hospice & Palliative CareCenter, 151

Hospice and Palliative Care, 65, 133, 140, 145

Hospice and Palliative Nurses Association, 145

Hospice care, *See also* Palliative care
    community hospice agencies, 133–147
    Department of Veterans Affairs programs, 35–36
    development of, 59
    eligibility criteria, 67
    history of programs in the Department of Veterans Affairs, 59–68
    Medicare Hospice Benefit, 36, 59, 61, 62, 138–139
    payment for, 35, 36
    stoicism and, 11–14

Hospice Education Network, 145

Hospice of Marin, 59, 62

The Hospice Movement, 61

Hospice Program Guide, 63

Hospice-Veteran Partnerships, 66, 133–147

Hostile environments
    Posttraumatic Stress Disorder and, 74–75

HPNA. *See* Hospice and Palliative Nurses Association

HVP. *See* Hospice-Veteran Partnerships

Hydrocodone, 122

Hydromorphone, 122

I

IASP. *See* International Association for the Study of Pain

Immigration Act of 1965, 50

Independence
    stoicism and, 12–13

International Association for the Study of Pain, 112

International Classification of Diseases, 223

Interprofessional Palliative Care Fellowship, 65

Iraq War
culture of combat, 28–29
demographics of surviving families, 191–192
demographics of the deceased, 190–191
statistics from, 27

"Irritable heart," 72

J

Joint Commission, 63

Jones, Diane, 66

K

Killed-in-action deaths, 200

Korean War
culture of combat, 8, 28
noncombat military deaths, 11
Silent Generation and, 49–50
statistics from, 27
Veterans Service Organization, 178, 183

L

Letter writing, therapeutic, 99

Lidocaine patches, 118

Life review, 78–81

Lou Gehrig's disease, 52

M

MacArthur, General Douglas, 50

Marijuana, 242

Marine Corps
culture of, 6

Masking, 220

McGill Pain Questionnaire, 112

Me Generation, 52

Media attention, 202

Medicare
Hospice Benefit, 36, 59, 61, 62, 138–139
veteran enrollment, 33, 135

Memorials
combat deaths and, 200–201
role in grief and loss, 161–168

Meperidine, 122

Mercy Care, 151–152

Methadone, 116

Military culture
commonalities of, 3, 48–52
culture of combat, 7–11
factors effecting, 26
hospice care delivery and, 19–23
stoicism and, 11–14
subculture of Posttraumatic Stress Disorder, 14–15
suicide and, 219–220
survivalists, 127–130

Military funerals
combat deaths and, 200–201
disruption of, 171–172, 202
enhancing the value of, 164–165
therapeutic value of, 162–164

Military History Checklist, 52, 144, 245

Military personnel. See also Military culture; Veterans
effectiveness of indoctrination, 6
effects of service on families, 5–6
feelings concerning military training, 4–5
impact of discharge from military, 5, 6–7
impact of service on identity, 25–26
reasons for joining the military, 3–4

Montreal Royal Victoria Palliative Care Service, 60

Moral distress
guilt and, 95
Posttraumatic Stress Disorder and, 72

Morphine sulfate, 122

Mount, Dr. Balfour, 60

N

Narcotics Anonymous, 117

Narrative Exposure Therapy, 79–80

Narrative Therapy, 79–80

National Cemetery Administration, 136

National Child Traumatic Stress Network, 201

National Hospice and Palliative Care Organization, 66, 140, 149, 181

National Hospice Study, 59

National Leadership Board, 67

National Vietnam Veterans Art Museum, 9

NCA. See National Cemetery Administration

Neuropathic pain, 111

"Neurosis," 72

NHPCO. See National Hospice and Palliative Care Organization

Nociceptive pain, 111

Non-Steroidal Anti-Inflammatory Drugs, 118–119

Notification of death, 198–199

NSAIDs. *See* Non-Steroidal Anti-Inflammatory Drugs

Numeric Rating Scale, 112

O

OAA. *See* Office of Academic Affiliations

OEF. *See* Operation Enduring Freedom

Office of Academic Affiliations, 64, 65

Office of Decedent Affairs, 178

Office of Geriatrics and Extended Care, 64, 65, 66

Ohio State Veterans Home, 105

OIF. *See* Operation Iraqi Freedom

Operation Enduring Freedom
culture of combat, 28–29
demographics of surviving families, 191–192
demographics of the deceased, 190–191
statistics from, 27

Operation Iraqi Freedom
culture of combat, 28–29
demographics of surviving families, 191–192
demographics of the deceased, 190–191
statistics from, 27

Opioids
abuse of, 116
adverse effects in some veterans with Posttraumatic
Stress Disorder, 120
instituting therapy, 121
opioid equivalency table, 122
side effects of, 119

Outpatient Palliative Care, 138

Oxycodone, 122

P

PADD. *See* Person authorized to direct disposition of
remains

Pain Disability Scale, 112

Pain management
adverse effects of opioids in some veterans with
Posttraumatic Stress Disorder, 120
instituting opioid therapy, 121
interaction between pain and Posttraumatic Stress
Disorder, 115–116
nonpharmacologic therapy, 117–118
opioid equivalency table, 122
pain assessment, 112–113
pain ladder, 121
persistent pain treatment, 117
pharmacologic therapy, 118–122

Posttraumatic Stress Disorder and, 114–116
prescription drug abuse, 116
stoicism and, 113–116
terminology, 111
treatment, 117–122
veteran culture and, 113–116

Palliative care. *See also* Hospice care
development of, 59
history of programs in the Department of Veterans
Affairs, 59–68
Outpatient Palliative Care, 138

Palliative Care Clinics, 138

Palliative Care Consult Team Directive, 138

Palliative Care Nursing Assistants, 145

Palliative Care Programs, 138

Palliative Treatment Program, 59

Palo Alto Health Care System, 61

Patriot Guard Riders, 171–172, 202

PCCT. *See* Palliative Care Consult Team Directive

PCNA. *See* Palliative Care Nursing Assistants

*Peace at Last: Stories of Hope and Healing for Veterans
and Their Families*, 105, 177

Persian Gulf War
culture of combat, 28
statistics from, 27

Person authorized to direct disposition of remains, 195

Phelps, Fred, 171–172

Pikes Peak Hospice & Palliative Care, 150–151

PNOK. *See* Primary Next of Kin

Posttraumatic Stress Disorder
adverse effects of opioids, 120
context of grieving prior to traumatic events, 86–89
coping with intense emotions, 80–81
counseling services, 90–91
delayed-onset, 76
exposure to violence trauma, 75–76
family grief and, 177–179, 194
grief as the root of traumatic stress, 89–90
grief support and, 182–183
hostile environment trauma, 74–75
incidence of, 76
interaction with pain, 115–116
life review, 78–81
military culture and, 14–15
moral distress and, 72
pain management and, 114–116
prescription drug abuse, 116
refusal of treatment, 12
secondary traumatization, 226–227
spiritual distress and, 73–74
suicide and, 224–226
symptoms, 72, 76
theoretical guidance, 79–80

trauma and, 71–72
treatment, 76–77
undiagnosed, 31

Postvention principles, 228–230

Prescription drug abuse
Posttraumatic Stress Disorder and, 116

Pride
stoicism and, 12–13

Primary Family Caregiver Benefits, 180

Primary Next of Kin, 192, 195, 201

Print resources, 244

Professional resources, 244

Pseudoaddictive behavior, 115

Psycho-education, 206

Psychotherapy, 79–80, 90–91, 117

PTP. *See* Palliative Treatment Program

PTSD. *See* Posttraumatic Stress Disorder

R

Readjustment Counseling Division, 91

Reconciliation rituals, 167

Rehabilitative care, 34

Religious beliefs, 32, 73–74

Respect for American Fallen Heroes Act, 171

Riley, Matilda White, 47

Rituals
combat deaths and, 200–201
role in grief and loss, 161–168

Robert Wood Johnson Foundation, 64

Roos, Louise, 179

S

Saunders, Cicely, 59, 60–61, 183

"Scatter bed" models, 61–62

Secondary Next of Kin, 192, 195

Secondary traumatization, 226–227

Selective serotonin re-uptake inhibitors, 120

Self blame, 87–89

Self-help groups, 206

Servicemen's Readjustment Act of 1944, 49

"Shell shock," 72

Shneidman, E., 233

Silent Generation, 48–50

SNOK. *See* Secondary Next of Kin

Somatic pain, 111

SOS. *See* Survivor Outreach Services Program

Spiritual issues, 32, 73–74

SSRIs. See Selective serotonin re-uptake inhibitors

St. Christopher's Hospice, 59

"Stand Downs," 135

State Veteran Service Officers, 143

State Veterans Homes, 142, 183–184

Steen, Ken, 213–217

Stein Hospice, 105

Stoicism
components of, 12–13
confusion with courage, 12
control and, 12–13
definition of, 11
grief and, 175, 181–182
importance for soldiers, 12, 13
independence and, 12–13
learning to let go of, 14
military culture and, 11–14
pain management and, 113–116

Suboxone, 116

Suicide
Army suicide behavior surveillance, 231
counseling military survivors, 231–234
dissembling, 220
ecological model, 220
impact on families, 226–227
masking, 220
military culture and, 219–220
military factors, 234–235
military policies and procedures, 230–231
military suicide statistics, 222–224
Posttraumatic Stress Disorder and, 224–226
predictors of, 224
principles of postvention, 228–230
secondary traumatization, 226–227
secret keeping and, 222
suicide notes, 221–222
survivors of, 227–228
system model, 220–228

Suicide postvention. Health promotion, risk reduction, and suicide prevention, 230

Support groups, 206

Survivalists, 127–130

Survivor benefits, 34

Survivor Outreach Services Program, 200, 207

Survivor's guilt, 96

SVH. See State Veterans Homes

T

TAPC. *See* Training and Program Assessment for Palliative Care

TAPS. *See* Tragedy Assistance Program for Survivors

TBI. *See* Traumatic Brain Injury

TCAs. *See* Tricyclic antidepressants

Therapeutic letter writing, 99

Therapeutic rituals, 166–168

Traditional Generation, 48–49

Tragedy Assistance Program for Survivors, 185, 200, 201, 207

Training and Program Assessment for Palliative Care, 64–66, 67

Transition rituals, 166–167

Trauma
    combat deaths and, 192–195
    counseling services, 90–91
    exposure to violence, 75–76
    hostile environment trauma, 74–75
    interrelationship with grief, 86–90
    Posttraumatic Stress Disorder and, 71–72

Traumatic Brain Injury, 225

Treating Specialty Code 96, 67

Tricyclic antidepressants, 119

Tuskegee Syphilis Study, 49

U

Uniform Benefits Package, 135

U.S. Department of Defense
    grief counseling, 91

U.S. Department of Veterans Affairs
    accountability requirements, 140
    available services, 34, 90–91
    Bereaved Family Survey, 145–146
    Central Office, 59–60
    characteristics of veterans enrolled at time of death, 33
    Community Based Outpatient Clinics, 34, 90, 138
    counseling services, 90–91
    culture of, 139
    enrollment information, 35
    funding for, 140
    Greater Los Angeles Health Care System, 61
    healthcare coverage, 35–36
    history of hospice and palliative care, 59–68
    Hospice and Palliative Care, 65, 133, 140, 145
    hospice service, 35–36, 138–139
    Hospice-Veteran Partnerships, 66, 133–147
    Office of Academic Affiliations, 64, 65
    Office of Decedent Affairs, 178
    Office of Geriatrics and Extended Care, 64, 65, 66
    Readjustment Counseling Division, 91
    role of, 32–34, 139–140
    unenrolled veterans, 35
    Uniform Benefits Package, 135
    VA Hospice and Palliative Care initiative, 65, 133, 140
    VA Medical Centers, 90, 137
    Vet Centers, 90–91, 138, 185, 205, 207
    We Honor Veterans, 140–141, 149–154
    websites, 35, 90

U.S. Marine Corps
    culture of, 6

V

VA. *See* U.S. Department of Veterans Affairs

VA Hospice and Palliative Care initiative, 66, 67

VA Medical Centers, 90, 137

VAHPC. *See* VA Hospice and Palliative Care initiative

VAMCs. *See* VA Medical Centers

VBA. *See* Veteran Benefits offices

VERA. *See* Veterans Equitable Resource Allocation System

Vet Centers, 90–91, 138, 185, 205, 207

Vet-to-Vet program, 136

Veteran Benefits offices, 90, 136

Veteran Outreach Centers. *See* Vet Centers

Veteran service organizations, 90

Veterans. *See also* Military culture; Military personnel; U.S. Department of Veterans Affairs
    annual death statistics, 29
    characteristics of enrolled in VA at time of death, 33
    clinical needs of, 30–32
    counseling services for, 85–92
    definition of, 143–144
    demographics, 29–30
    end-of-life care decisions, 135
    generational cohorts, 47–52
    homeless, 135
    resources, 243–244
    service related medical conditions, 39–43
    special issues with end of life treatment, 55 56
    spiritual issues, 32
    ways to support, 32

Veterans Equitable Resource Allocation System, 63

Veterans Health Administration, 34, 135, 136–138

Veterans Health Administration Directive, 67

Veterans Health Care Eligibility Act of 1996, 63

Veterans History Project, 11, 153

Veterans Integrated Service Networks, 137

Veterans of Foreign Wars, 10–11, 90, 136, 142–143

Veterans' Service Organizations, 136, 142–143, 178, 183

VHA. *See* Veterans Health Administration

Vietnam Veterans Memorial, 99, 167

Vietnam War
Agent Orange related medical conditions, 40–43
Baby Boomer Generation and, 50–51
culture of combat, 9–11, 28
noncombat military deaths, 11
statistics from, 27

Violence
Posttraumatic Stress Disorder and, 75–76

Visceral pain, 111

VISNs. *See* Veterans Integrated Service Networks

VITAS Innovative Hospice Care of Atlanta Metro, 153–154

Volunteers, 152–153

VSOs. *See* Veteran service organizations

W

Wadsworth program, 59–60

War memorials
role in grief and loss, 162, 165–166

We Honor Veterans, 140–141, 149–154

Websites
American Association of Suicidology, 233
Army grief support services, 207
Bereaved Family Survey, 146
caregiver support, 180
Department of Veterans Affairs, 90
Department of Veterans Affairs enrollment
information, 35
grief resources, 243
military family resources, 244
print resources, 244
professional resources, 244
Vet Centers, 207
veteran resources, 243–244
Veterans History Project, 11
Veterans Service Organizations, 143
We Honor Veterans, 149

Westboro Baptist Church, 171–172

WHO. *See* World Health Organization

WHV. *See We Honor Veterans*

Widows, military, 213–217

Wind-up pain, 111

World Health Organization, 118, 121

World War II
American Soldier Study, 241

culture of combat, 8, 10, 27–28
GI Generation and, 49
statistics from, 27

Wounded Warriors: Their Last Battle, 181